Women's Wellness Journal and Log Book

Women's Wellness Journal and Log Book: Six Month Women's Health and Fitness Journal

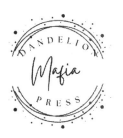

How do I use this journal?

The short answer is: HOWEVER YOU WANT.

This women's wellness journal is all about YOU and your wellness. So you get to decide how to use it, what to focus on, and the goals you set out for yourself.

This journal and log book covers 6 months, so you can take things slow to start, and add wellness habits as you go, or you can commit to tracking everything listed each day from the beginning.

The thing is though, this journal has to be used as a tool for your growth, and it's important that you allow the journal to be an extension of your wellness practices, not a nagging pressure-pusher.

There are symbols that accompany almost every prompt. Feel free to shade in the appropriate symbol to represent completion as you go through your journal each day. If desired, use the lines for written reflection and self-understanding.

There are also lots of blank spaces in the margins to add whatever you want. Doodle if that's your thing!

I hope this journal will help you see your beauty and power, and will be an incredible tool in your development.

xo, Shannon

Taking Care of Body.

DATE: _____   S M T W T F S

TODAY'S GOALS

MEALS

	CALORIES	FAT	PROTEIN	CARBS
BREAKFAST				
LUNCH				
DINNER				
SNACKS				

HYDRATION

SUPPLEMENTS
☺

HOURS SLEPT LAST NIGHT
Z Z Z Z Z Z Z +

EXERCISE

	TIME	DISTANCE	WEIGHT	REPS	SETS
ACTIVITY 1					
ACTIVITY 2					
ACTIVITY 3					
ACTIVITY 4					

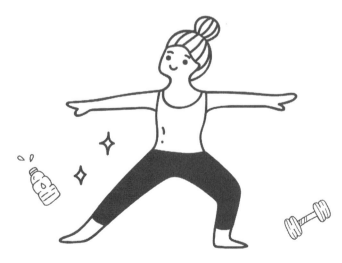

Mind & Spirit

PRAYER/MEDITATION 🙏

Reflections:

_____

_____

_____

_____

SELF - CARE 🖤

I looked after me by:

_____

_____

_____

_____

GRATITUDE ⭐

I am grateful for:

_____

_____

_____

_____

TODAY I FEEL 😲 🙂 😢 😐 😠

_____

_____

Taking Care of Body,

DATE: _____   S M T W T F S

TODAY'S GOALS

MEALS

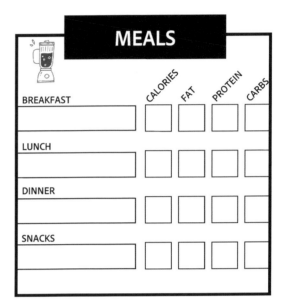

	CALORIES	FAT	PROTEIN	CARBS
BREAKFAST				
LUNCH				
DINNER				
SNACKS				

HYDRATION

SUPPLEMENTS

☺

HOURS SLEPT LAST NIGHT

ZZZZZZZ +

EXERCISE

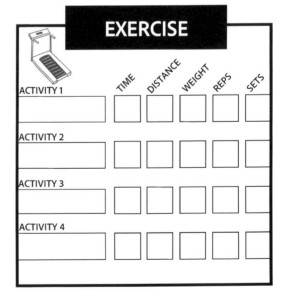

	TIME	DISTANCE	WEIGHT	REPS	SETS
ACTIVITY 1					
ACTIVITY 2					
ACTIVITY 3					
ACTIVITY 4					

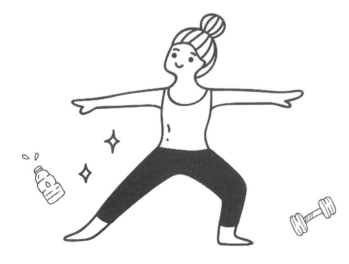

Mind & Spirit

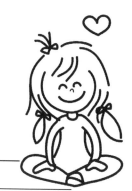

PRAYER/MEDITATION 🙏

Reflections:

_____

_____

_____

SELF - CARE ♥

I looked after me by:

_____

_____

_____

GRATITUDE ⭐

I am grateful for:

_____

_____

_____

TODAY I FEEL 😲 🙂 😢 😐 😠

_____

_____

Taking Care of Body,

DATE: _____   S M T W T F S

TODAY'S GOALS

MEALS

	CALORIES	FAT	PROTEIN	CARBS
BREAKFAST				
LUNCH				
DINNER				
SNACKS				

HYDRATION

SUPPLEMENTS

☺

HOURS SLEPT LAST NIGHT

Z Z Z Z Z Z Z +

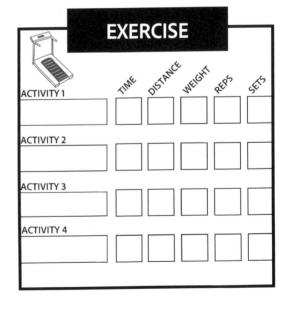

EXERCISE

	TIME	DISTANCE	WEIGHT	REPS	SETS
ACTIVITY 1					
ACTIVITY 2					
ACTIVITY 3					
ACTIVITY 4					

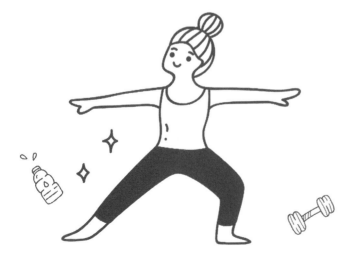

Mind & Spirit

PRAYER/MEDITATION 🙏

Reflections: _____

_____

_____

_____

SELF - CARE ❤️

I looked after me by: _____

_____

_____

_____

GRATITUDE ⭐

I am grateful for: _____

_____

_____

_____

TODAY I FEEL 😮 🙂 🥺 😐 😡

_____

_____

Taking Care of Body,

DATE: _____   S M T W T F S

TODAY'S GOALS

MEALS

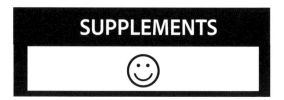

	CALORIES	FAT	PROTEIN	CARBS
BREAKFAST				
LUNCH				
DINNER				
SNACKS				

HYDRATION

SUPPLEMENTS

☺

HOURS SLEPT LAST NIGHT

Z Z Z Z Z Z Z +

EXERCISE

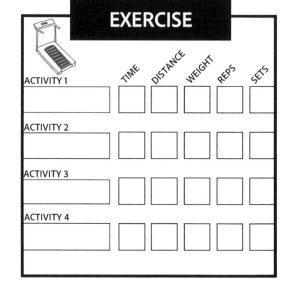

	TIME	DISTANCE	WEIGHT	REPS	SETS
ACTIVITY 1					
ACTIVITY 2					
ACTIVITY 3					
ACTIVITY 4					

Mind & Spirit

PRAYER/MEDITATION 🙏

Reflections:

_____

_____

_____

_____

SELF - CARE 💜

I looked after me by:

_____

_____

_____

_____

GRATITUDE ⭐

I am grateful for:

_____

_____

_____

_____

TODAY I FEEL 😲 🙂 😢 😐 😠

_____

_____

Taking Care of Body

DATE: _____   **S M T W T F S**

TODAY'S GOALS

MEALS

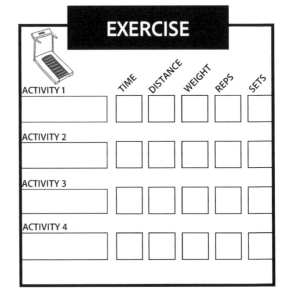

	CALORIES	FAT	PROTEIN	CARBS
BREAKFAST				
LUNCH				
DINNER				
SNACKS				

HYDRATION

SUPPLEMENTS

:)

HOURS SLEPT LAST NIGHT

Z Z Z Z Z Z Z Z +

EXERCISE

	TIME	DISTANCE	WEIGHT	REPS	SETS
ACTIVITY 1					
ACTIVITY 2					
ACTIVITY 3					
ACTIVITY 4					

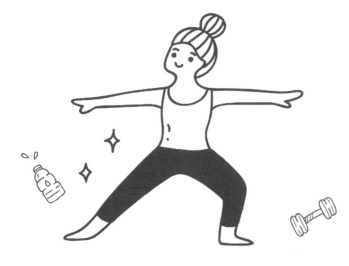

Mind & Spirit

PRAYER/MEDITATION 🙏

Reflections:

_____

_____

_____

_____

SELF - CARE 🖤

I looked after me by:

_____

_____

_____

_____

GRATITUDE ⭐

I am grateful for:

_____

_____

_____

_____

TODAY I FEEL 😮 🙂 😢 😐 😠

_____

_____

Taking Care of Body,

DATE: _____   S M T W T F S

TODAY'S GOALS

MEALS

	CALORIES	FAT	PROTEIN	CARBS
BREAKFAST				
LUNCH				
DINNER				
SNACKS				

HYDRATION

SUPPLEMENTS

:)

HOURS SLEPT LAST NIGHT

ZZZZZZZ+

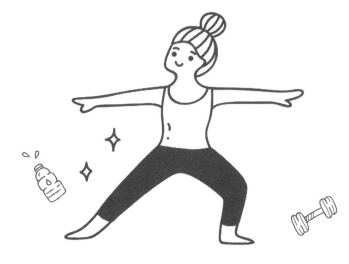

EXERCISE

	TIME	DISTANCE	WEIGHT	REPS	SETS
ACTIVITY 1					
ACTIVITY 2					
ACTIVITY 3					
ACTIVITY 4					

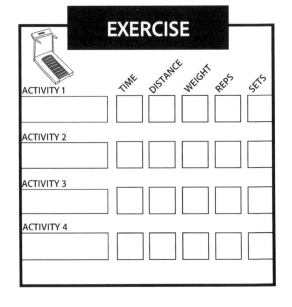

Mind & Spirit

PRAYER/MEDITATION 🙏

Reflections:

_____

_____

_____

SELF - CARE ♥

I looked after me by:

_____

_____

_____

GRATITUDE ✦

I am grateful for:

_____

_____

_____

TODAY I FEEL 😮 🙂 🥺 😐 😠

_____

_____

Taking Care of Body,

DATE: [_____]   S M T W T F S

TODAY'S GOALS

MEALS

	CALORIES	FAT	PROTEIN	CARBS
BREAKFAST				
LUNCH				
DINNER				
SNACKS				

HYDRATION

SUPPLEMENTS

☺

HOURS SLEPT LAST NIGHT

Z Z Z Z Z Z Z +

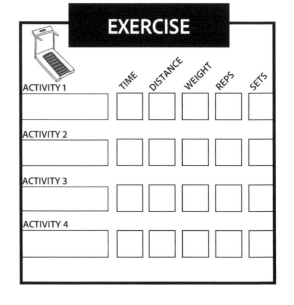

EXERCISE

	TIME	DISTANCE	WEIGHT	REPS	SETS
ACTIVITY 1					
ACTIVITY 2					
ACTIVITY 3					
ACTIVITY 4					

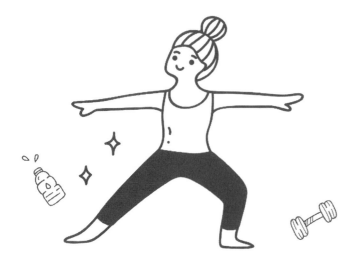

Mind & Spirit

PRAYER/MEDITATION 🙏

Reflections:

_____

_____

_____

SELF - CARE 🤍

I looked after me by:

_____

_____

_____

GRATITUDE ⭐

I am grateful for:

_____

_____

_____

TODAY I FEEL 😮 🙂 😢 😐 😠

_____

_____

Taking Care of Body,

DATE: _____   S M T W T F S

TODAY'S GOALS

MEALS

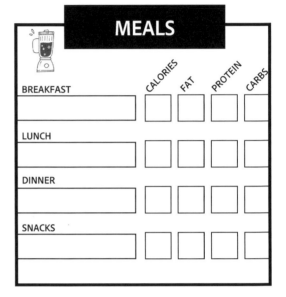

	CALORIES	FAT	PROTEIN	CARBS
BREAKFAST				
LUNCH				
DINNER				
SNACKS				

HYDRATION

[cup] [cup] [cup] [cup] [cup] [cup] [cup] [cup]

SUPPLEMENTS

☺

HOURS SLEPT LAST NIGHT

Z Z Z Z Z Z Z +

EXERCISE

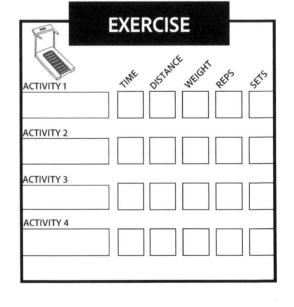

	TIME	DISTANCE	WEIGHT	REPS	SETS
ACTIVITY 1					
ACTIVITY 2					
ACTIVITY 3					
ACTIVITY 4					

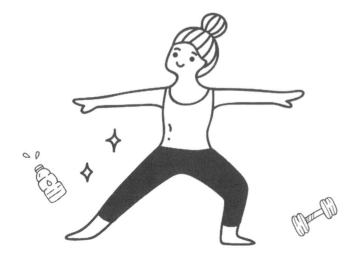

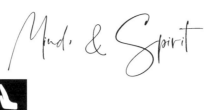

PRAYER/MEDITATION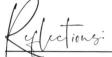

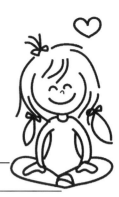

Reflections: _____
_____
_____
_____

SELF - CARE ♥

I looked after me by: _____
_____
_____
_____

GRATITUDE ⭐

I am grateful for: _____
_____
_____
_____

TODAY I FEEL 😲 🙂 😢 😐 😠

_____
_____

Taking Care of Body

TODAY'S GOALS

MEALS

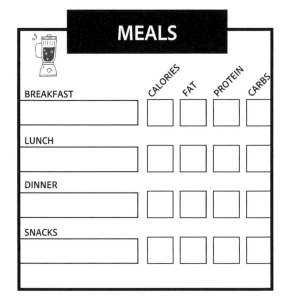

	CALORIES	FAT	PROTEIN	CARBS
BREAKFAST				
LUNCH				
DINNER				
SNACKS				

HYDRATION

SUPPLEMENTS

☺

HOURS SLEPT LAST NIGHT

Z Z Z Z Z Z Z Z +

EXERCISE

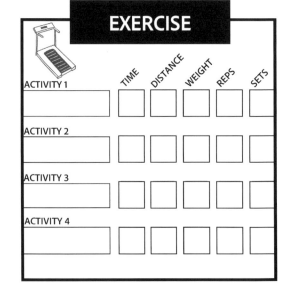

	TIME	DISTANCE	WEIGHT	REPS	SETS
ACTIVITY 1					
ACTIVITY 2					
ACTIVITY 3					
ACTIVITY 4					

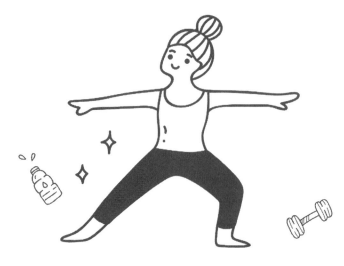

Mind & Spirit

PRAYER/MEDITATION 🙏

Reflections:

_____

_____

_____

_____

SELF - CARE 🖤

I looked after me by:

_____

_____

_____

_____

GRATITUDE ⭐

I am grateful for:

_____

_____

_____

_____

TODAY I FEEL 😲 🙂 😢 😐 😠

_____

_____

Taking Care of Body,

DATE: [_____] S M T W T F S

TODAY'S GOALS

MEALS

	CALORIES	FAT	PROTEIN	CARBS
BREAKFAST				
LUNCH				
DINNER				
SNACKS				

HYDRATION

SUPPLEMENTS

☺

HOURS SLEPT LAST NIGHT

Z Z Z Z Z Z Z +

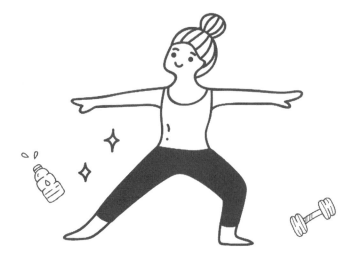

EXERCISE

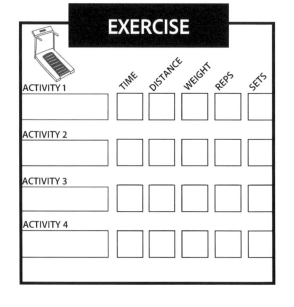

	TIME	DISTANCE	WEIGHT	REPS	SETS
ACTIVITY 1					
ACTIVITY 2					
ACTIVITY 3					
ACTIVITY 4					

Mind & Spirit

PRAYER/MEDITATION 🙏

Reflections:

_____

_____

_____

_____

SELF - CARE ♥

I looked after me by:

_____

_____

_____

_____

GRATITUDE ⭐

I am grateful for:

_____

_____

_____

_____

TODAY I FEEL 😮 🙂 🥺 😐 😠

_____

_____

Taking Care of Body.

DATE: _____   S M T W T F S

TODAY'S GOALS

MEALS

	CALORIES	FAT	PROTEIN	CARBS
BREAKFAST				
LUNCH				
DINNER				
SNACKS				

HYDRATION

SUPPLEMENTS

HOURS SLEPT LAST NIGHT

Z Z Z Z Z Z Z +

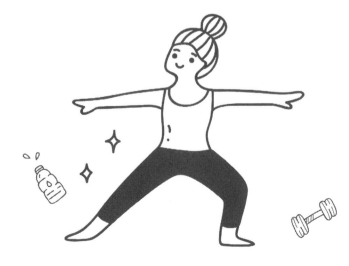

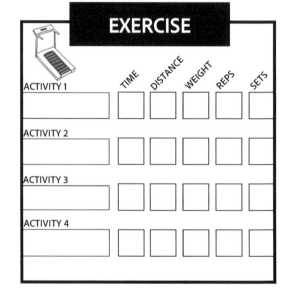

EXERCISE

	TIME	DISTANCE	WEIGHT	REPS	SETS
ACTIVITY 1					
ACTIVITY 2					
ACTIVITY 3					
ACTIVITY 4					

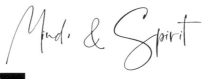

PRAYER/MEDITATION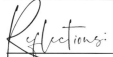

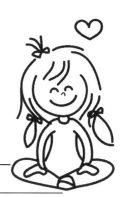

Reflections:

_____

_____

_____

SELF - CARE ♥

I looked after me by:

_____

_____

_____

GRATITUDE ✦

I am grateful for:

_____

_____

_____

TODAY I FEEL 😮 🙂 😢 😐 😠

_____

_____

Taking Care of Body,

DATE: _____   S M T W T F S

TODAY'S GOALS

MEALS

	CALORIES	FAT	PROTEIN	CARBS
BREAKFAST				
LUNCH				
DINNER				
SNACKS				

HYDRATION

SUPPLEMENTS

☺

HOURS SLEPT LAST NIGHT

ZZZZZZZ+

EXERCISE

	TIME	DISTANCE	WEIGHT	REPS	SETS
ACTIVITY 1					
ACTIVITY 2					
ACTIVITY 3					
ACTIVITY 4					

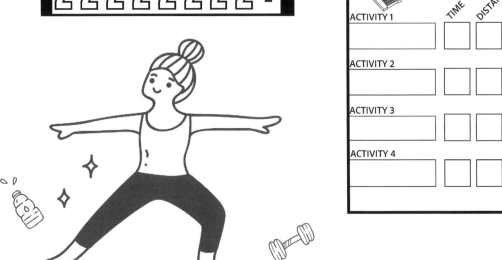

Mind & Spirit

PRAYER/MEDITATION 🙏

Reflections:

_____

_____

_____

_____

SELF - CARE 💜

I looked after me by:

_____

_____

_____

_____

GRATITUDE ⭐

I am grateful for:

_____

_____

_____

_____

TODAY I FEEL 😲 🙂 😢 😐 😠

_____

_____

Taking Care of Body,

DATE: _____   S M T W T F S

TODAY'S GOALS

MEALS

	CALORIES	FAT	PROTEIN	CARBS
BREAKFAST				
LUNCH				
DINNER				
SNACKS				

HYDRATION

SUPPLEMENTS
☺

HOURS SLEPT LAST NIGHT
ZZZZZZZ+

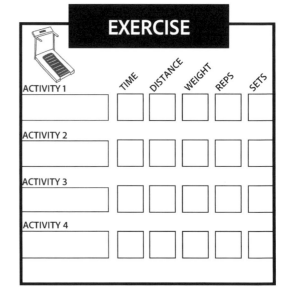

EXERCISE

	TIME	DISTANCE	WEIGHT	REPS	SETS
ACTIVITY 1					
ACTIVITY 2					
ACTIVITY 3					
ACTIVITY 4					

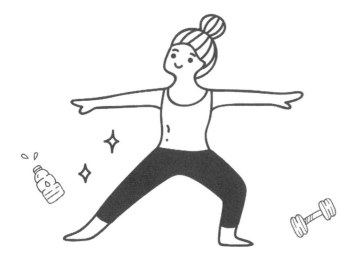

Mind & Spirit

PRAYER/MEDITATION 🙏

Reflections:

_____
_____
_____

SELF - CARE ♥

I looked after me by:

_____
_____
_____

GRATITUDE ⭐

I am grateful for:

_____
_____
_____

TODAY I FEEL 😲 🙂 😢 😐 😠

_____
_____

Taking Care of Body.

DATE: _____   S M T W T F S

TODAY'S GOALS

MEALS

	CALORIES	FAT	PROTEIN	CARBS
BREAKFAST				
LUNCH				
DINNER				
SNACKS				

HYDRATION

SUPPLEMENTS

☺

HOURS SLEPT LAST NIGHT

Z Z Z Z Z Z Z ✚

EXERCISE

	TIME	DISTANCE	WEIGHT	REPS	SETS
ACTIVITY 1					
ACTIVITY 2					
ACTIVITY 3					
ACTIVITY 4					

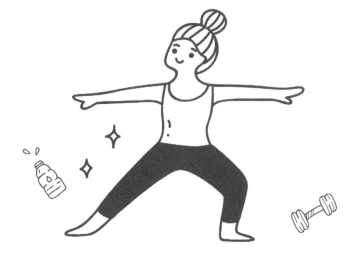

Mind & Spirit

PRAYER/MEDITATION 🙏

Reflections:

_____

_____

_____

_____

SELF - CARE 🖤

I looked after me by:

_____

_____

_____

_____

GRATITUDE ⭐

I am grateful for:

_____

_____

_____

_____

TODAY I FEEL 😲 🙂 😢 😐 😠

_____

_____

Taking Care of Body,

DATE: _____   S M T W T F S

TODAY'S GOALS

MEALS

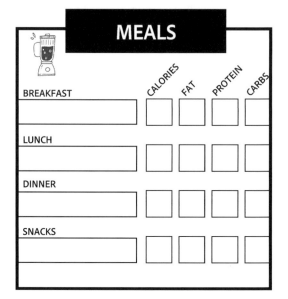

	CALORIES	FAT	PROTEIN	CARBS
BREAKFAST				
LUNCH				
DINNER				
SNACKS				

HYDRATION

SUPPLEMENTS

☺

HOURS SLEPT LAST NIGHT

ZZZZZZZ+

EXERCISE

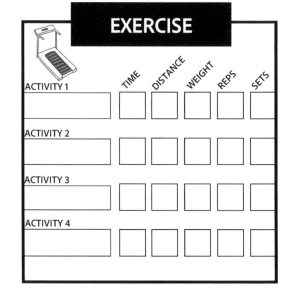

	TIME	DISTANCE	WEIGHT	REPS	SETS
ACTIVITY 1					
ACTIVITY 2					
ACTIVITY 3					
ACTIVITY 4					

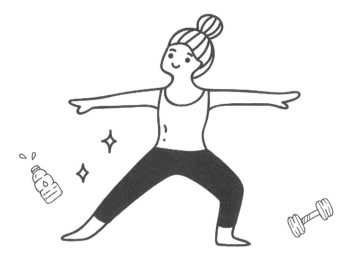

Mind & Spirit

PRAYER/MEDITATION

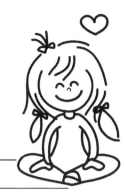

Reflections:

_____

_____

_____

_____

SELF - CARE ♥

I looked after me by:

_____

_____

_____

_____

GRATITUDE ✦

I am grateful for:

_____

_____

_____

_____

TODAY I FEEL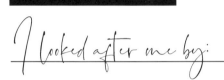

_____

_____

Taking Care of Body,

DATE: _____   S M T W T F S

TODAY'S GOALS

MEALS

	CALORIES	FAT	PROTEIN	CARBS
BREAKFAST				
LUNCH				
DINNER				
SNACKS				

HYDRATION

SUPPLEMENTS

☺

HOURS SLEPT LAST NIGHT

Z Z Z Z Z Z Z +

EXERCISE

	TIME	DISTANCE	WEIGHT	REPS	SETS
ACTIVITY 1					
ACTIVITY 2					
ACTIVITY 3					
ACTIVITY 4					

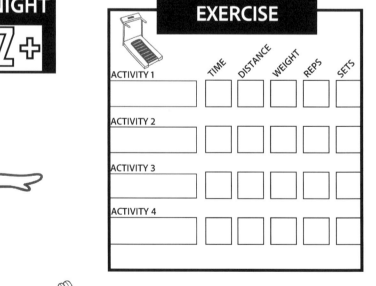

Mind & Spirit

PRAYER/MEDITATION 🙏

Reflections:

_____

_____

_____

_____

SELF - CARE 💛

I looked after me by:

_____

_____

_____

_____

GRATITUDE ⭐

I am grateful for:

_____

_____

_____

_____

TODAY I FEEL 😲 🙂 😢 😐 😠

_____

_____

Taking Care of Body

DATE: _____   S M T W T F S

TODAY'S GOALS

MEALS

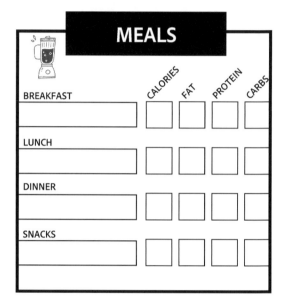

	CALORIES	FAT	PROTEIN	CARBS
BREAKFAST				
LUNCH				
DINNER				
SNACKS				

HYDRATION

◻◻◻◻◻◻◻◻

SUPPLEMENTS

☺

HOURS SLEPT LAST NIGHT

Z Z Z Z Z Z Z +

EXERCISE

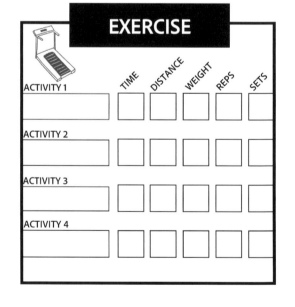

	TIME	DISTANCE	WEIGHT	REPS	SETS
ACTIVITY 1					
ACTIVITY 2					
ACTIVITY 3					
ACTIVITY 4					

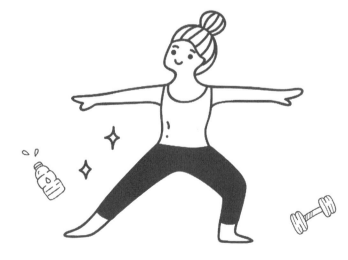

Mind & Spirit

PRAYER/MEDITATION 🙏

Reflections:

_____

_____

_____

SELF - CARE 🖤

I looked after me by:

_____

_____

_____

GRATITUDE ⭐

I am grateful for:

_____

_____

_____

TODAY I FEEL 😮 🙂 😢 😐 😠

_____

_____

Taking Care of Body

DATE: _____   S M T W T F S

TODAY'S GOALS

MEALS

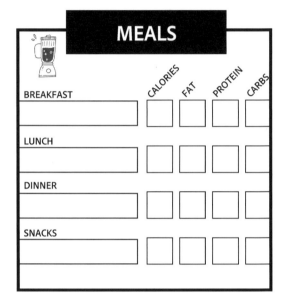

	CALORIES	FAT	PROTEIN	CARBS
BREAKFAST				
LUNCH				
DINNER				
SNACKS				

HYDRATION

SUPPLEMENTS

☺

HOURS SLEPT LAST NIGHT

ZZZZZZZ+

EXERCISE

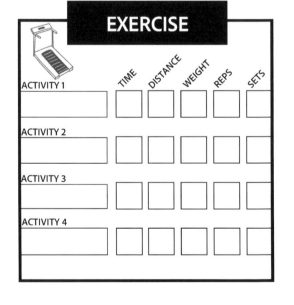

	TIME	DISTANCE	WEIGHT	REPS	SETS
ACTIVITY 1					
ACTIVITY 2					
ACTIVITY 3					
ACTIVITY 4					

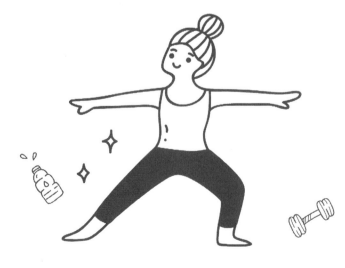

Mind & Spirit

PRAYER/MEDITATION 🙏

Reflections:

_____
_____
_____
_____

SELF - CARE 🖤

I looked after me by:

_____
_____
_____
_____

GRATITUDE ⭐

I am grateful for:

_____
_____
_____
_____

TODAY I FEEL 😮 🙂 😢 😐 😠

_____
_____

Taking Care of Body

TODAY'S GOALS

MEALS

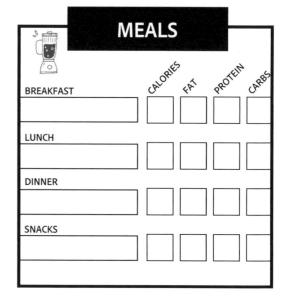

	CALORIES	FAT	PROTEIN	CARBS
BREAKFAST				
LUNCH				
DINNER				
SNACKS				

HYDRATION

SUPPLEMENTS

☺

HOURS SLEPT LAST NIGHT

Z Z Z Z Z Z Z +

EXERCISE

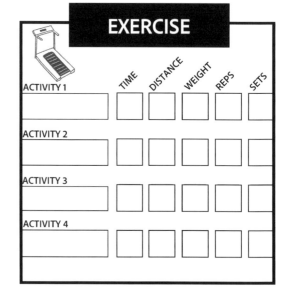

	TIME	DISTANCE	WEIGHT	REPS	SETS
ACTIVITY 1					
ACTIVITY 2					
ACTIVITY 3					
ACTIVITY 4					

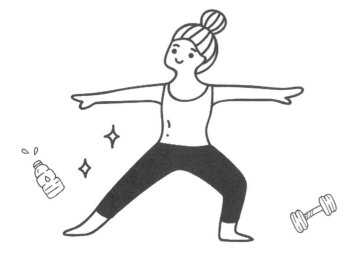

Mind & Spirit

PRAYER/MEDITATION 🙏

Reflections:

_____

_____

_____

_____

SELF - CARE ♥

I looked after me by:

_____

_____

_____

_____

GRATITUDE ⭐

I am grateful for:

_____

_____

_____

_____

TODAY I FEEL 😮 🙂 😢 😐 😠

_____

_____

Taking Care of Body,

DATE: _____   S M T W T F S

TODAY'S GOALS

MEALS

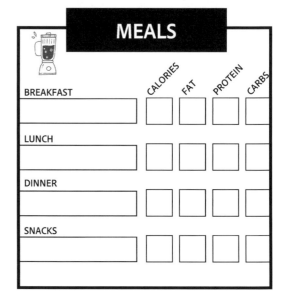

	CALORIES	FAT	PROTEIN	CARBS
BREAKFAST				
LUNCH				
DINNER				
SNACKS				

HYDRATION

SUPPLEMENTS

☺

HOURS SLEPT LAST NIGHT

ZZZZZZZ +

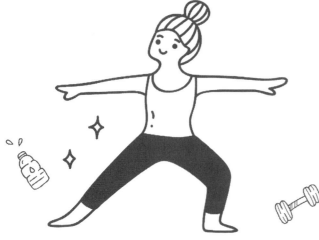

EXERCISE

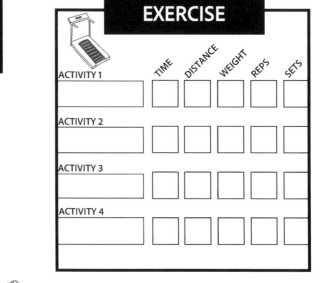

	TIME	DISTANCE	WEIGHT	REPS	SETS
ACTIVITY 1					
ACTIVITY 2					
ACTIVITY 3					
ACTIVITY 4					

Mind & Spirit

PRAYER/MEDITATION 🙏

Reflections:

_____

_____

_____

_____

SELF - CARE 💚

I looked after me by:

_____

_____

_____

_____

GRATITUDE ⭐

I am grateful for:

_____

_____

_____

_____

TODAY I FEEL 😮 🙂 😢 😐 😠

_____

_____

Taking Care of Body,

DATE: _____   **S M T W T F S**

TODAY'S GOALS

MEALS

	CALORIES	FAT	PROTEIN	CARBS
BREAKFAST				
LUNCH				
DINNER				
SNACKS				

HYDRATION

SUPPLEMENTS

☺

HOURS SLEPT LAST NIGHT

Z Z Z Z Z Z Z +

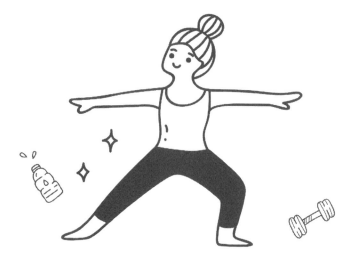

EXERCISE

	TIME	DISTANCE	WEIGHT	REPS	SETS
ACTIVITY 1					
ACTIVITY 2					
ACTIVITY 3					
ACTIVITY 4					

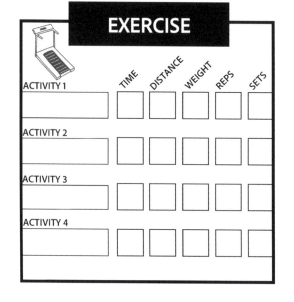

Mind & Spirit

PRAYER/MEDITATION 🙏

Reflections:

_____

_____

_____

_____

SELF - CARE ♥

I looked after me by:

_____

_____

_____

_____

GRATITUDE ⭐

I am grateful for:

_____

_____

_____

_____

TODAY I FEEL 😮 🙂 😢 😐 😠

_____

_____

Taking Care of Body

DATE: _____   S M T W T F S

TODAY'S GOALS

MEALS

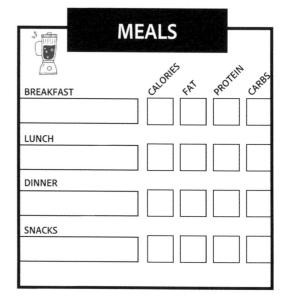

	CALORIES	FAT	PROTEIN	CARBS
BREAKFAST				
LUNCH				
DINNER				
SNACKS				

HYDRATION

SUPPLEMENTS

☺

HOURS SLEPT LAST NIGHT

ZZZZZZZ+

EXERCISE

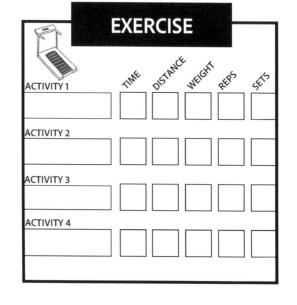

	TIME	DISTANCE	WEIGHT	REPS	SETS
ACTIVITY 1					
ACTIVITY 2					
ACTIVITY 3					
ACTIVITY 4					

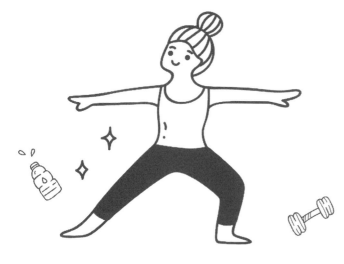

Mind & Spirit

PRAYER/MEDITATION 🙏

Reflections:

_____

_____

_____

_____

SELF - CARE ♥

I looked after me by:

_____

_____

_____

_____

GRATITUDE ⭐

I am grateful for:

_____

_____

_____

_____

TODAY I FEEL 😮 🙂 😢 😐 😠

_____

_____

Taking Care of Body

DATE: _____   S M T W T F S

TODAY'S GOALS

MEALS

	CALORIES	FAT	PROTEIN	CARBS
BREAKFAST				
LUNCH				
DINNER				
SNACKS				

HYDRATION

SUPPLEMENTS

🙂

HOURS SLEPT LAST NIGHT

ZZZZZZZ+

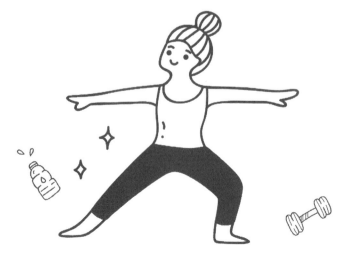

EXERCISE

	TIME	DISTANCE	WEIGHT	REPS	SETS
ACTIVITY 1					
ACTIVITY 2					
ACTIVITY 3					
ACTIVITY 4					

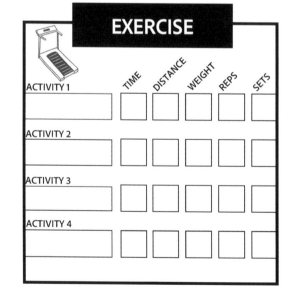

Mind & Spirit

PRAYER/MEDITATION 🙏

Reflections:

_____
_____
_____
_____

SELF - CARE 🖤

I looked after me by:

_____
_____
_____
_____

GRATITUDE ✪

I am grateful for:

_____
_____
_____
_____

TODAY I FEEL 😮 🙂 😢 😐 😠

_____
_____

Taking Care of Body,

DATE: _____   **S M T W T F S**

TODAY'S GOALS

(blank lined list)

MEALS

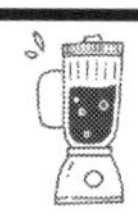

	CALORIES	FAT	PROTEIN	CARBS
BREAKFAST				
LUNCH				
DINNER				
SNACKS				

HYDRATION

▭ ▭ ▭ ▭ ▭ ▭ ▭ ▭

SUPPLEMENTS

☺

HOURS SLEPT LAST NIGHT

Z Z Z Z Z Z Z +

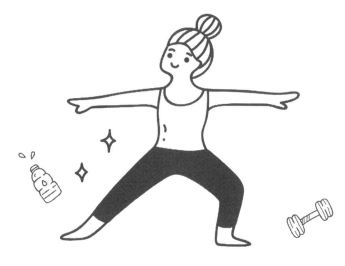

EXERCISE

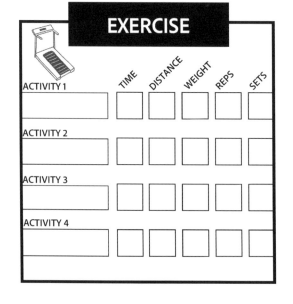

	TIME	DISTANCE	WEIGHT	REPS	SETS
ACTIVITY 1					
ACTIVITY 2					
ACTIVITY 3					
ACTIVITY 4					

Mind & Spirit

PRAYER/MEDITATION 🙏

Reflections: _____

_____

_____

_____

SELF - CARE 🖤

I looked after me by: _____

_____

_____

_____

GRATITUDE ⭐

I am grateful for: _____

_____

_____

_____

TODAY I FEEL 😲 🙂 😢 😐 😠

_____

_____

Taking Care of Body,

DATE: _____   **S M T W T F S**

TODAY'S GOALS

MEALS

	CALORIES	FAT	PROTEIN	CARBS
BREAKFAST				
LUNCH				
DINNER				
SNACKS				

HYDRATION

SUPPLEMENTS

☺

HOURS SLEPT LAST NIGHT

ZZZZZZZ +

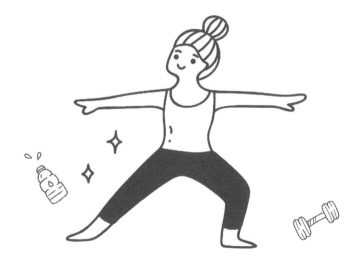

EXERCISE

	TIME	DISTANCE	WEIGHT	REPS	SETS
ACTIVITY 1					
ACTIVITY 2					
ACTIVITY 3					
ACTIVITY 4					

Mind & Spirit

PRAYER/MEDITATION 🙏

Reflections:

_____
_____
_____
_____

SELF - CARE 🖤

I looked after me by:

_____
_____
_____
_____

GRATITUDE ⭐

I am grateful for:

_____
_____
_____
_____

TODAY I FEEL 😮 🙂 😢 😐 😠

_____
_____

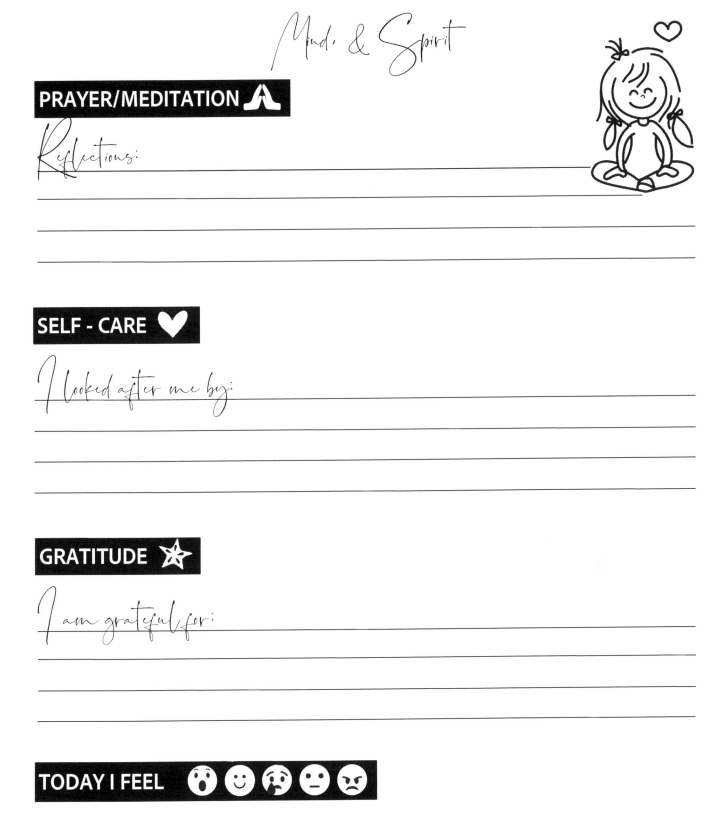

Taking Care of Body,

DATE: [_____]   S M T W T F S

TODAY'S GOALS

MEALS

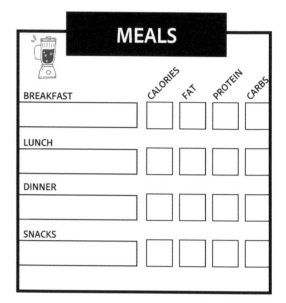

	CALORIES	FAT	PROTEIN	CARBS
BREAKFAST				
LUNCH				
DINNER				
SNACKS				

HYDRATION

SUPPLEMENTS

☺

HOURS SLEPT LAST NIGHT

Z Z Z Z Z Z Z +

EXERCISE

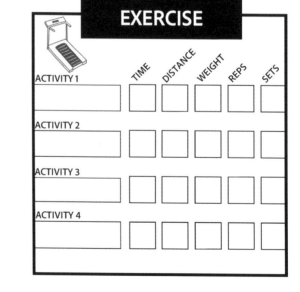

	TIME	DISTANCE	WEIGHT	REPS	SETS
ACTIVITY 1					
ACTIVITY 2					
ACTIVITY 3					
ACTIVITY 4					

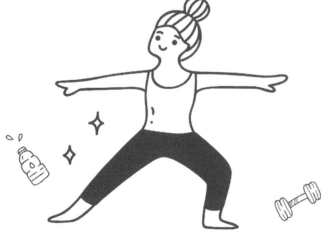

Mind & Spirit

PRAYER/MEDITATION 🙏

Reflections:

_____
_____
_____
_____

SELF - CARE ♥

I looked after me by:

_____
_____
_____
_____

GRATITUDE ⭐

I am grateful for:

_____
_____
_____
_____

TODAY I FEEL 😮 🙂 😢 😐 😠

_____
_____

Taking Care of Body,

DATE: _____   S M T W T F S

TODAY'S GOALS

MEALS

	CALORIES	FAT	PROTEIN	CARBS
BREAKFAST				
LUNCH				
DINNER				
SNACKS				

HYDRATION

SUPPLEMENTS

☺

HOURS SLEPT LAST NIGHT

ZZZZZZZ+

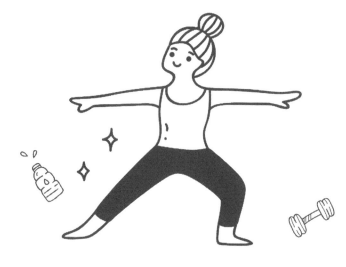

EXERCISE

	TIME	DISTANCE	WEIGHT	REPS	SETS
ACTIVITY 1					
ACTIVITY 2					
ACTIVITY 3					
ACTIVITY 4					

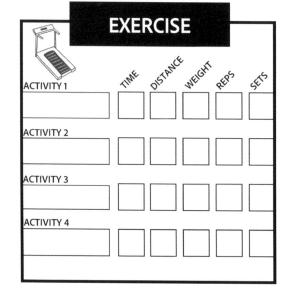

Mind & Spirit

PRAYER/MEDITATION 🙏

Reflections:

_____

_____

_____

_____

SELF - CARE 💜

I looked after me by:

_____

_____

_____

_____

GRATITUDE ⭐

I am grateful for:

_____

_____

_____

_____

TODAY I FEEL 😲 🙂 😢 😐 😠

_____

_____

Taking Care of Body,

DATE: _____   S M T W T F S

TODAY'S GOALS

MEALS

	CALORIES	FAT	PROTEIN	CARBS
BREAKFAST				
LUNCH				
DINNER				
SNACKS				

HYDRATION

SUPPLEMENTS

🙂

HOURS SLEPT LAST NIGHT

Z Z Z Z Z Z Z +

EXERCISE

	TIME	DISTANCE	WEIGHT	REPS	SETS
ACTIVITY 1					
ACTIVITY 2					
ACTIVITY 3					
ACTIVITY 4					

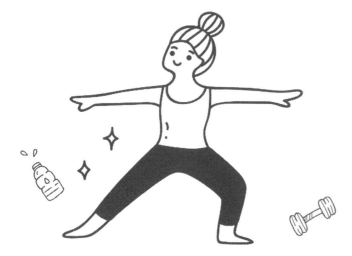

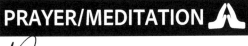 Mind & Spirit

PRAYER/MEDITATION 🙏

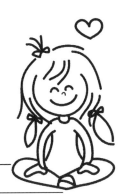

Reflections:

_____

_____

_____

_____

SELF - CARE ♥

I looked after me by:

_____

_____

_____

_____

GRATITUDE ⭐

I am grateful for:

_____

_____

_____

_____

TODAY I FEEL 😮 🙂 😢 😐 😠

_____

_____

Taking Care of Body

DATE: _____   S M T W T F S

TODAY'S GOALS

MEALS

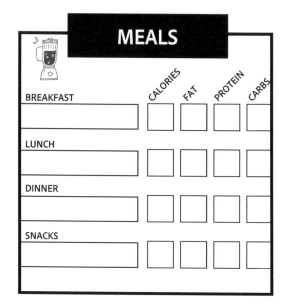

	CALORIES	FAT	PROTEIN	CARBS
BREAKFAST				
LUNCH				
DINNER				
SNACKS				

HYDRATION

🥤 🥤 🥤 🥤 🥤 🥤 🥤 🥤

SUPPLEMENTS

☺

HOURS SLEPT LAST NIGHT

Z Z Z Z Z Z Z +

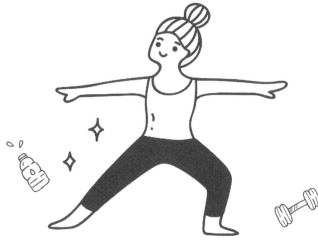

EXERCISE

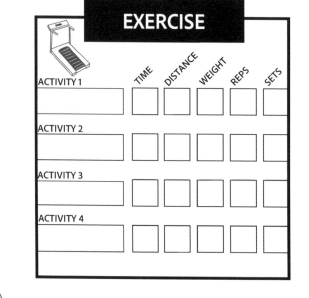

	TIME	DISTANCE	WEIGHT	REPS	SETS
ACTIVITY 1					
ACTIVITY 2					
ACTIVITY 3					
ACTIVITY 4					

Mind & Spirit

PRAYER/MEDITATION 🙏

Reflections:

_____
_____
_____
_____

SELF - CARE 🖤

I looked after me by:

_____
_____
_____
_____

GRATITUDE ⭐

I am grateful for:

_____
_____
_____
_____

TODAY I FEEL 😮 🙂 😢 😐 😠

_____
_____

Taking Care of Body

DATE: _____   S M T W T F S

TODAY'S GOALS

MEALS

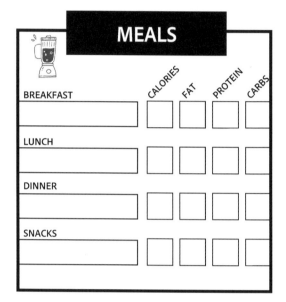

	CALORIES	FAT	PROTEIN	CARBS
BREAKFAST				
LUNCH				
DINNER				
SNACKS				

HYDRATION

SUPPLEMENTS

☺

HOURS SLEPT LAST NIGHT

Z Z Z Z Z Z Z +

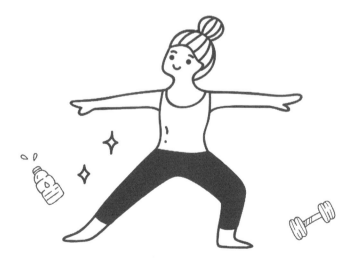

EXERCISE

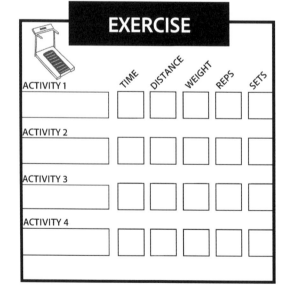

	TIME	DISTANCE	WEIGHT	REPS	SETS
ACTIVITY 1					
ACTIVITY 2					
ACTIVITY 3					
ACTIVITY 4					

Mind & Spirit

PRAYER/MEDITATION 🙏

Reflections:

_____
_____
_____
_____

SELF - CARE 🖤

I looked after me by:

_____
_____
_____
_____

GRATITUDE ⭐

I am grateful for:

_____
_____
_____
_____

TODAY I FEEL 😮 🙂 😢 😐 😠

_____
_____

Taking Care of Body

DATE: [_____]   S M T W T F S

TODAY'S GOALS

(blank lined list)

MEALS

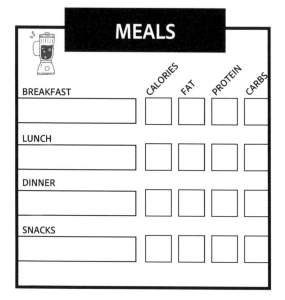

	CALORIES	FAT	PROTEIN	CARBS
BREAKFAST				
LUNCH				
DINNER				
SNACKS				

HYDRATION

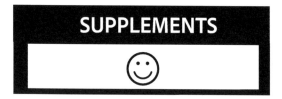

SUPPLEMENTS

☺

HOURS SLEPT LAST NIGHT

Z Z Z Z Z Z Z +

EXERCISE

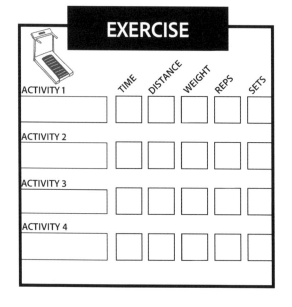

	TIME	DISTANCE	WEIGHT	REPS	SETS
ACTIVITY 1					
ACTIVITY 2					
ACTIVITY 3					
ACTIVITY 4					

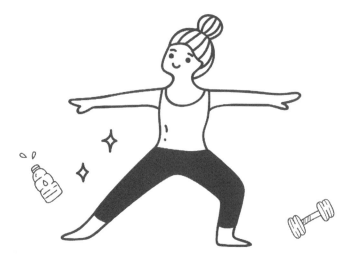

Mind & Spirit

PRAYER/MEDITATION 🙏

Reflections:

_____

_____

_____

_____

SELF - CARE ♥

I looked after me by:

_____

_____

_____

_____

GRATITUDE ⭐

I am grateful for:

_____

_____

_____

_____

TODAY I FEEL 😲 🙂 😢 😐 😠

_____

_____

Taking Care of Body

DATE: _____   **S M T W T F S**

TODAY'S GOALS

_____
_____
_____
_____
_____
_____
_____
_____

MEALS

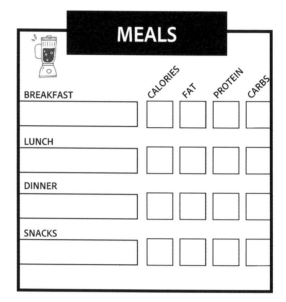

	CALORIES	FAT	PROTEIN	CARBS
BREAKFAST				
LUNCH				
DINNER				
SNACKS				

HYDRATION

SUPPLEMENTS

☺

HOURS SLEPT LAST NIGHT

Z Z Z Z Z Z Z +

EXERCISE

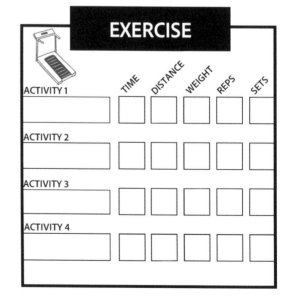

	TIME	DISTANCE	WEIGHT	REPS	SETS
ACTIVITY 1					
ACTIVITY 2					
ACTIVITY 3					
ACTIVITY 4					

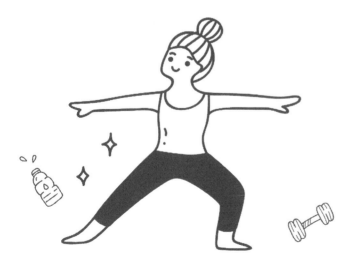

Mind & Spirit

PRAYER/MEDITATION 🙏

Reflections:

_____

_____

_____

_____

SELF - CARE 🖤

I looked after me by:

_____

_____

_____

_____

GRATITUDE ⭐

I am grateful for:

_____

_____

_____

_____

TODAY I FEEL 😲 🙂 😢 😐 😠

_____

_____

Taking Care of Body,

DATE: _____   S M T W T F S

TODAY'S GOALS

MEALS

	CALORIES	FAT	PROTEIN	CARBS
BREAKFAST				
LUNCH				
DINNER				
SNACKS				

HYDRATION

SUPPLEMENTS

☺

HOURS SLEPT LAST NIGHT

Z Z Z Z Z Z Z +

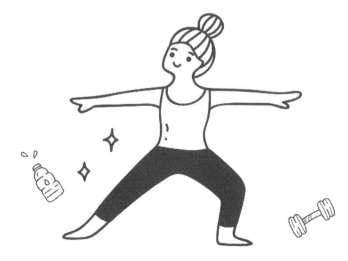

EXERCISE

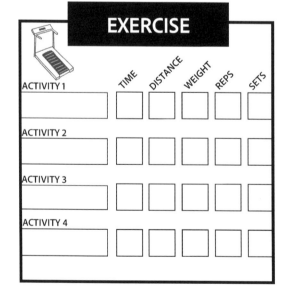

	TIME	DISTANCE	WEIGHT	REPS	SETS
ACTIVITY 1					
ACTIVITY 2					
ACTIVITY 3					
ACTIVITY 4					

Mind & Spirit

PRAYER/MEDITATION 🙏

Reflections: _____

_____

_____

_____

SELF - CARE 🖤

I looked after me by: _____

_____

_____

_____

GRATITUDE ⭐

I am grateful for: _____

_____

_____

_____

TODAY I FEEL 😮 🙂 😢 😐 😠

_____

_____

Taking Care of Body,

DATE: _____   S M T W T F S

TODAY'S GOALS

MEALS

	CALORIES	FAT	PROTEIN	CARBS
BREAKFAST				
LUNCH				
DINNER				
SNACKS				

HYDRATION

SUPPLEMENTS

☺

HOURS SLEPT LAST NIGHT

Z Z Z Z Z Z Z +

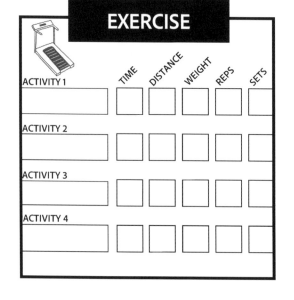

EXERCISE

	TIME	DISTANCE	WEIGHT	REPS	SETS
ACTIVITY 1					
ACTIVITY 2					
ACTIVITY 3					
ACTIVITY 4					

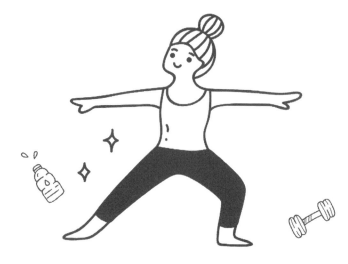

Mind & Spirit

PRAYER/MEDITATION 🙏

Reflections: _____

_____

_____

_____

SELF - CARE 🖤

I looked after me by: _____

_____

_____

_____

GRATITUDE ⭐

I am grateful for: _____

_____

_____

_____

TODAY I FEEL 😲 🙂 😢 😐 😠

_____

_____

Taking Care of Body

DATE: _____   **S M T W T F S**

TODAY'S GOALS

MEALS

	CALORIES	FAT	PROTEIN	CARBS
BREAKFAST				
LUNCH				
DINNER				
SNACKS				

HYDRATION

SUPPLEMENTS

☺

HOURS SLEPT LAST NIGHT

Z Z Z Z Z Z Z +

EXERCISE

	TIME	DISTANCE	WEIGHT	REPS	SETS
ACTIVITY 1					
ACTIVITY 2					
ACTIVITY 3					
ACTIVITY 4					

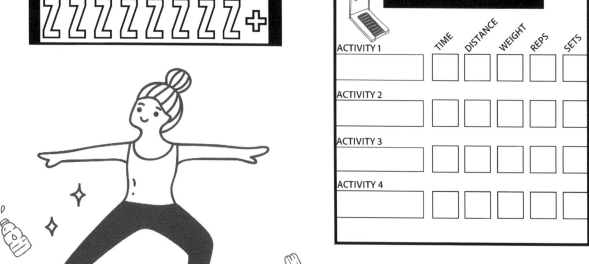

Mind & Spirit

PRAYER/MEDITATION 🙏

Reflections:

_____
_____
_____
_____

SELF - CARE 💙

I looked after me by:

_____
_____
_____
_____

GRATITUDE ⭐

I am grateful for:

_____
_____
_____
_____

TODAY I FEEL 😮 🙂 😢 😐 😠

_____
_____

Taking Care of Body,

DATE: _____   S M T W T F S

TODAY'S GOALS

MEALS

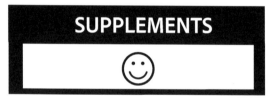

	CALORIES	FAT	PROTEIN	CARBS
BREAKFAST				
LUNCH				
DINNER				
SNACKS				

HYDRATION

SUPPLEMENTS

☺

HOURS SLEPT LAST NIGHT

Z Z Z Z Z Z Z +

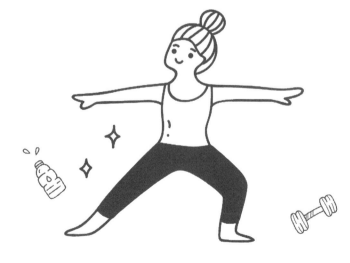

EXERCISE

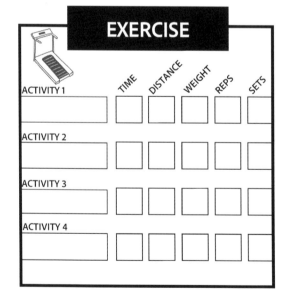

	TIME	DISTANCE	WEIGHT	REPS	SETS
ACTIVITY 1					
ACTIVITY 2					
ACTIVITY 3					
ACTIVITY 4					

Mind & Spirit

PRAYER/MEDITATION 🙏

Reflections:

_____

_____

_____

SELF - CARE ♥

I looked after me by:

_____

_____

_____

GRATITUDE ⭐

I am grateful for:

_____

_____

_____

TODAY I FEEL 😮 🙂 😢 😐 😠

_____

_____

Taking Care of Body,

DATE: _____   **S M T W T F S**

TODAY'S GOALS

MEALS

	CALORIES	FAT	PROTEIN	CARBS
BREAKFAST				
LUNCH				
DINNER				
SNACKS				

HYDRATION

SUPPLEMENTS

☺

HOURS SLEPT LAST NIGHT

Z Z Z Z Z Z Z +

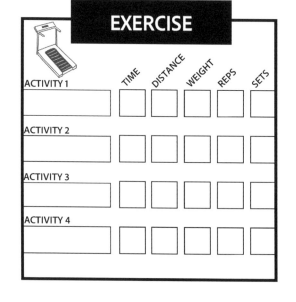

EXERCISE

	TIME	DISTANCE	WEIGHT	REPS	SETS
ACTIVITY 1					
ACTIVITY 2					
ACTIVITY 3					
ACTIVITY 4					

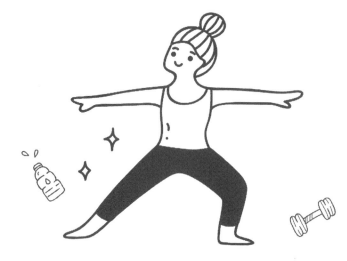

Mind & Spirit

PRAYER/MEDITATION 🙏

Reflections:

_____
_____
_____
_____

SELF - CARE 💛

I looked after me by:

_____
_____
_____
_____

GRATITUDE ⭐

I am grateful for:

_____
_____
_____
_____

TODAY I FEEL 😲 🙂 😢 😐 😠

_____
_____

Taking Care of Body,

DATE: _____ S M T W T F S

TODAY'S GOALS

MEALS

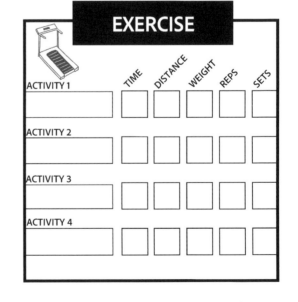

	CALORIES	FAT	PROTEIN	CARBS
BREAKFAST				
LUNCH				
DINNER				
SNACKS				

HYDRATION

SUPPLEMENTS

☺

HOURS SLEPT LAST NIGHT

Z Z Z Z Z Z Z +

EXERCISE

	TIME	DISTANCE	WEIGHT	REPS	SETS
ACTIVITY 1					
ACTIVITY 2					
ACTIVITY 3					
ACTIVITY 4					

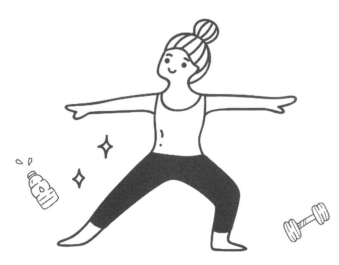

Mind & Spirit

PRAYER/MEDITATION 🙏

Reflections:

_____

_____

_____

SELF - CARE ♥

I looked after me by:

_____

_____

_____

GRATITUDE ⭐

I am grateful for:

_____

_____

_____

TODAY I FEEL 😮 🙂 😢 😐 😡

_____

_____

Taking Care of Body

TODAY'S GOALS

MEALS

	CALORIES	FAT	PROTEIN	CARBS
BREAKFAST				
LUNCH				
DINNER				
SNACKS				

HYDRATION

SUPPLEMENTS

☺

HOURS SLEPT LAST NIGHT

Z Z Z Z Z Z Z +

EXERCISE

	TIME	DISTANCE	WEIGHT	REPS	SETS
ACTIVITY 1					
ACTIVITY 2					
ACTIVITY 3					
ACTIVITY 4					

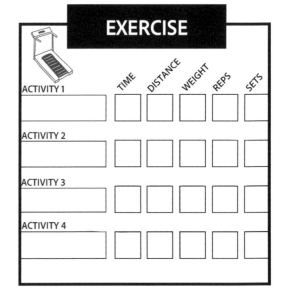

Mind & Spirit

PRAYER/MEDITATION 🙏

Reflections:

_____
_____
_____

SELF - CARE 🖤

I looked after me by:

_____
_____
_____

GRATITUDE ⭐

I am grateful for:

_____
_____
_____

TODAY I FEEL 😮 🙂 😢 😐 😠

_____
_____

Taking Care of Body,

DATE: _____   S M T W T F S

TODAY'S GOALS

_____
_____
_____
_____
_____
_____
_____
_____
_____

MEALS

	CALORIES	FAT	PROTEIN	CARBS
BREAKFAST				
LUNCH				
DINNER				
SNACKS				

HYDRATION

SUPPLEMENTS

HOURS SLEPT LAST NIGHT
Z Z Z Z Z Z Z +

EXERCISE

	TIME	DISTANCE	WEIGHT	REPS	SETS
ACTIVITY 1					
ACTIVITY 2					
ACTIVITY 3					
ACTIVITY 4					

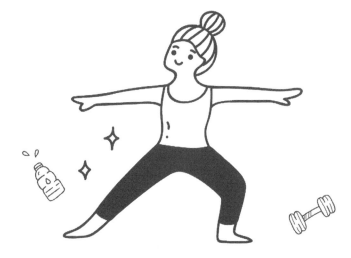

Mind & Spirit

PRAYER/MEDITATION 🙏

Reflections:

_____
_____
_____
_____

SELF - CARE 💜

I looked after me by:

_____
_____
_____
_____

GRATITUDE ⭐

I am grateful for:

_____
_____
_____
_____

TODAY I FEEL 😲 🙂 😢 😐 😠

_____
_____

Taking Care of Body,

DATE: [   ]   S M T W T F S

TODAY'S GOALS

MEALS

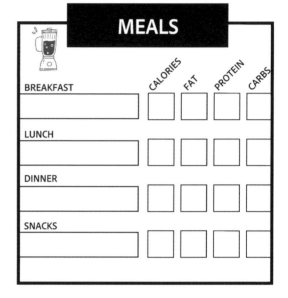

	CALORIES	FAT	PROTEIN	CARBS
BREAKFAST				
LUNCH				
DINNER				
SNACKS				

HYDRATION

SUPPLEMENTS

☺

HOURS SLEPT LAST NIGHT

Z Z Z Z Z Z Z +

EXERCISE

	TIME	DISTANCE	WEIGHT	REPS	SETS
ACTIVITY 1					
ACTIVITY 2					
ACTIVITY 3					
ACTIVITY 4					

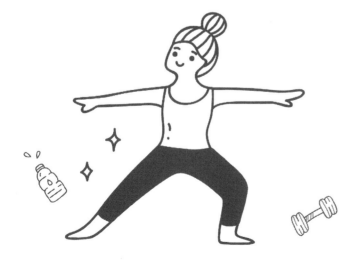

Mind & Spirit

PRAYER/MEDITATION 🙏

Reflections:

_____
_____
_____
_____

SELF - CARE 🖤

I looked after me by:

_____
_____
_____

GRATITUDE ⭐

I am grateful for:

_____
_____
_____

TODAY I FEEL 😮 🙂 🥺 😐 😠

_____
_____

Taking Care of Body

DATE: _____   **S M T W T F S**

TODAY'S GOALS

MEALS

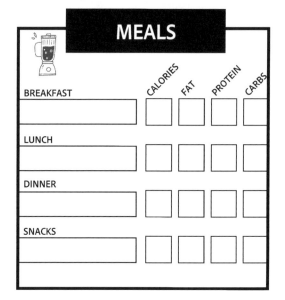

	CALORIES	FAT	PROTEIN	CARBS
BREAKFAST				
LUNCH				
DINNER				
SNACKS				

HYDRATION

SUPPLEMENTS

☺

HOURS SLEPT LAST NIGHT

Z Z Z Z Z Z Z ✚

EXERCISE

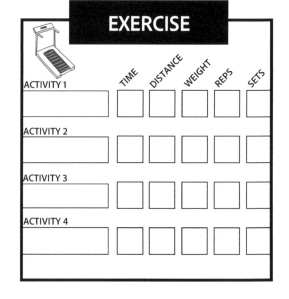

	TIME	DISTANCE	WEIGHT	REPS	SETS
ACTIVITY 1					
ACTIVITY 2					
ACTIVITY 3					
ACTIVITY 4					

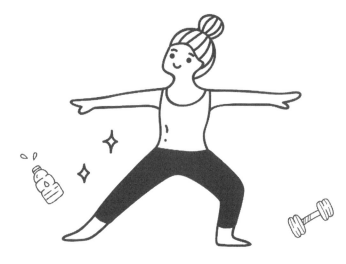

Mind & Spirit

PRAYER/MEDITATION 🙏

Reflections:

_____

_____

_____

SELF - CARE 🖤

I looked after me by:

_____

_____

_____

GRATITUDE ⭐

I am grateful for:

_____

_____

_____

TODAY I FEEL 😮 🙂 😢 😐 😠

_____

_____

Taking Care of Body,

DATE: _____   S M T W T F S

TODAY'S GOALS

MEALS

	CALORIES	FAT	PROTEIN	CARBS
BREAKFAST				
LUNCH				
DINNER				
SNACKS				

HYDRATION

SUPPLEMENTS

☺

HOURS SLEPT LAST NIGHT

Z Z Z Z Z Z Z +

EXERCISE

	TIME	DISTANCE	WEIGHT	REPS	SETS
ACTIVITY 1					
ACTIVITY 2					
ACTIVITY 3					
ACTIVITY 4					

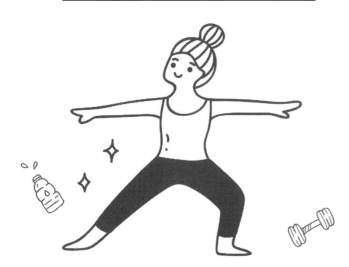

Mind & Spirit

PRAYER/MEDITATION 🙏

Reflections:

_____

_____

_____

SELF - CARE 🖤

I looked after me by:

_____

_____

_____

GRATITUDE ⭐

I am grateful for:

_____

_____

_____

TODAY I FEEL 😮 🙂 😢 😐 😠

_____

_____

Taking Care of Body.

DATE: [_____]   S M T W T F S

TODAY'S GOALS

MEALS

	CALORIES	FAT	PROTEIN	CARBS
BREAKFAST				
LUNCH				
DINNER				
SNACKS				

HYDRATION

SUPPLEMENTS

:)

HOURS SLEPT LAST NIGHT

ZZZZZZZ+

EXERCISE

	TIME	DISTANCE	WEIGHT	REPS	SETS
ACTIVITY 1					
ACTIVITY 2					
ACTIVITY 3					
ACTIVITY 4					

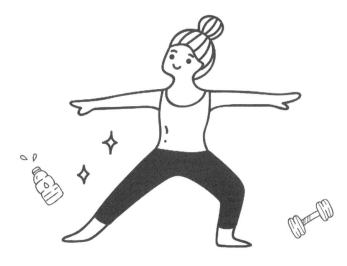
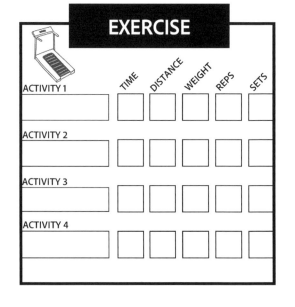

Mind & Spirit

PRAYER/MEDITATION 🙏

Reflections:

_____

_____

_____

SELF - CARE 🖤

I looked after me by:

_____

_____

_____

GRATITUDE ⭐

I am grateful for:

_____

_____

_____

TODAY I FEEL 😮 🙂 😢 😐 😠

_____

_____

Taking Care of Body.

DATE: _____   S M T W T F S

TODAY'S GOALS

MEALS

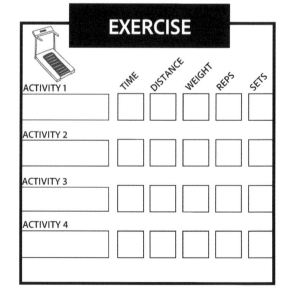

	CALORIES	FAT	PROTEIN	CARBS
BREAKFAST				
LUNCH				
DINNER				
SNACKS				

HYDRATION

SUPPLEMENTS

☺

HOURS SLEPT LAST NIGHT

Z Z Z Z Z Z Z +

EXERCISE

	TIME	DISTANCE	WEIGHT	REPS	SETS
ACTIVITY 1					
ACTIVITY 2					
ACTIVITY 3					
ACTIVITY 4					

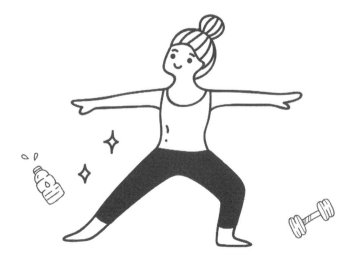

Mind & Spirit

PRAYER/MEDITATION 🙏

Reflections:

_____
_____
_____
_____

SELF - CARE 🖤

I looked after me by:

_____
_____
_____
_____

GRATITUDE ⭐

I am grateful for:

_____
_____
_____
_____

TODAY I FEEL 😮 🙂 😢 😐 😠

_____
_____

Taking Care of Body,

DATE: _____   **S M T W T F S**

TODAY'S GOALS

MEALS

	CALORIES	FAT	PROTEIN	CARBS
BREAKFAST				
LUNCH				
DINNER				
SNACKS				

HYDRATION

🥤 🥤 🥤 🥤 🥤 🥤 🥤 🥤

SUPPLEMENTS

☺

HOURS SLEPT LAST NIGHT

Z Z Z Z Z Z Z +

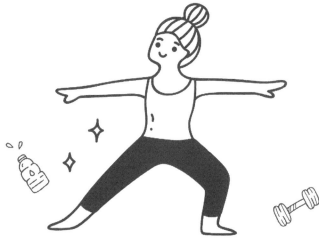

EXERCISE

	TIME	DISTANCE	WEIGHT	REPS	SETS
ACTIVITY 1					
ACTIVITY 2					
ACTIVITY 3					
ACTIVITY 4					

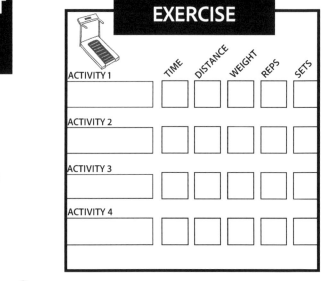

Mind & Spirit

PRAYER/MEDITATION 🙏
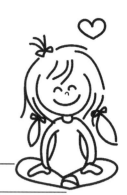

Reflections:

_____

_____

_____

SELF - CARE 💚

I looked after me by:

_____

_____

_____

GRATITUDE ⭐

I am grateful for:

_____

_____

_____

TODAY I FEEL 😮 🙂 😢 😐 😠

_____

_____

Taking Care of Body

DATE: _____   S M T W T F S

TODAY'S GOALS

MEALS

	CALORIES	FAT	PROTEIN	CARBS
BREAKFAST				
LUNCH				
DINNER				
SNACKS				

HYDRATION

SUPPLEMENTS

☺

HOURS SLEPT LAST NIGHT

Z Z Z Z Z Z Z +

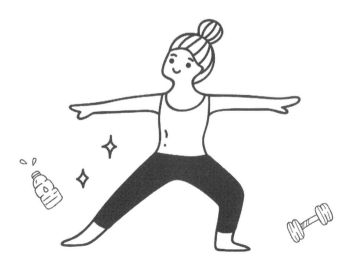

EXERCISE

	TIME	DISTANCE	WEIGHT	REPS	SETS
ACTIVITY 1					
ACTIVITY 2					
ACTIVITY 3					
ACTIVITY 4					

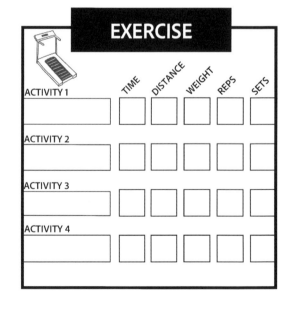

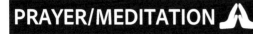

PRAYER/MEDITATION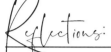

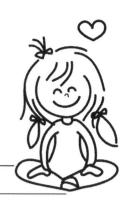

Reflections:

_____

_____

_____

SELF - CARE ♥

I looked after me by:

_____

_____

_____

GRATITUDE ⭐

I am grateful for:

_____

_____

_____

TODAY I FEEL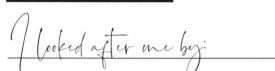

_____

_____

Taking Care of Body.

DATE: _____   S M T W T F S

TODAY'S GOALS

MEALS

	CALORIES	FAT	PROTEIN	CARBS
BREAKFAST				
LUNCH				
DINNER				
SNACKS				

HYDRATION

SUPPLEMENTS

☺

HOURS SLEPT LAST NIGHT

Z Z Z Z Z Z Z +

EXERCISE

	TIME	DISTANCE	WEIGHT	REPS	SETS
ACTIVITY 1					
ACTIVITY 2					
ACTIVITY 3					
ACTIVITY 4					

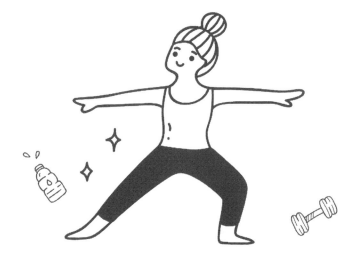

Mind & Spirit

PRAYER/MEDITATION 🙏

Reflections:

_____
_____
_____
_____

SELF - CARE 🖤

I looked after me by:

_____
_____
_____
_____

GRATITUDE ✦

I am grateful for:

_____
_____
_____
_____

TODAY I FEEL 😮 🙂 😢 😐 😠

_____
_____

Taking Care of Body.

DATE: _____   S M T W T F S

TODAY'S GOALS

MEALS

	CALORIES	FAT	PROTEIN	CARBS
BREAKFAST				
LUNCH				
DINNER				
SNACKS				

HYDRATION

SUPPLEMENTS

HOURS SLEPT LAST NIGHT

Z Z Z Z Z Z Z +

EXERCISE

	TIME	DISTANCE	WEIGHT	REPS	SETS
ACTIVITY 1					
ACTIVITY 2					
ACTIVITY 3					
ACTIVITY 4					

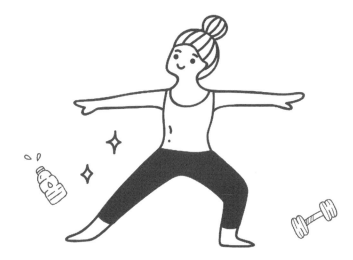

Mind & Spirit

PRAYER/MEDITATION 🙏

Reflections:

_____

_____

_____

_____

SELF - CARE 🖤

I looked after me by:

_____

_____

_____

_____

GRATITUDE ⭐

I am grateful for:

_____

_____

_____

_____

TODAY I FEEL 😮 🙂 😢 😐 😠

_____

_____

Taking Care of Body,

DATE: _____   S M T W T F S

TODAY'S GOALS

MEALS

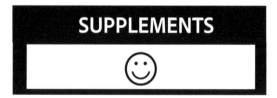

	CALORIES	FAT	PROTEIN	CARBS
BREAKFAST				
LUNCH				
DINNER				
SNACKS				

HYDRATION

SUPPLEMENTS

☺

HOURS SLEPT LAST NIGHT

ZZZZZZZ✛

EXERCISE

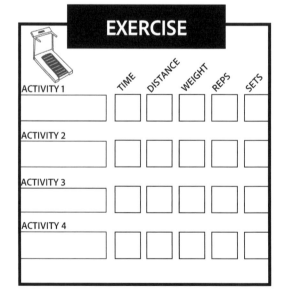

	TIME	DISTANCE	WEIGHT	REPS	SETS
ACTIVITY 1					
ACTIVITY 2					
ACTIVITY 3					
ACTIVITY 4					

Mind & Spirit

PRAYER/MEDITATION 🙏

Reflections:

_____
_____
_____

SELF - CARE 🖤

I looked after me by:

_____
_____
_____

GRATITUDE ⭐

I am grateful for:

_____
_____
_____

TODAY I FEEL 😮 🙂 😢 😐 😠

_____
_____

Taking Care of Body.

DATE: _____   S M T W T F S

TODAY'S GOALS

MEALS

	CALORIES	FAT	PROTEIN	CARBS
BREAKFAST				
LUNCH				
DINNER				
SNACKS				

HYDRATION

SUPPLEMENTS

☺

HOURS SLEPT LAST NIGHT

Z Z Z Z Z Z Z +

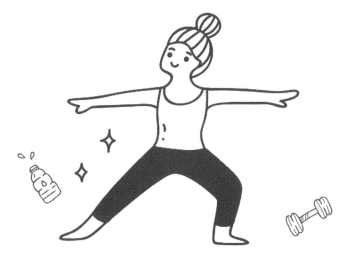

EXERCISE

	TIME	DISTANCE	WEIGHT	REPS	SETS
ACTIVITY 1					
ACTIVITY 2					
ACTIVITY 3					
ACTIVITY 4					

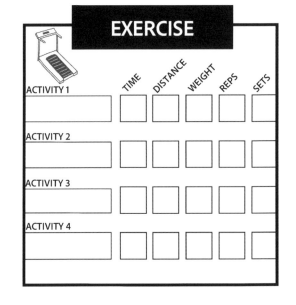

Mind & Spirit

PRAYER/MEDITATION 🙏

Reflections:

_____

_____

_____

_____

SELF - CARE 🖤

I looked after me by:

_____

_____

_____

_____

GRATITUDE ⭐

I am grateful for:

_____

_____

_____

_____

TODAY I FEEL 😮 🙂 😢 😐 😠

_____

_____

Taking Care of Body

DATE: _____

S M T W T F S

TODAY'S GOALS

(blank lined list)

MEALS

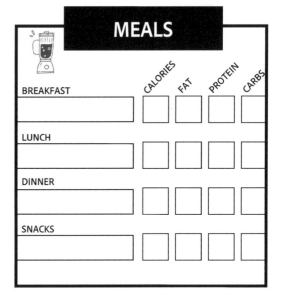

	CALORIES	FAT	PROTEIN	CARBS
BREAKFAST				
LUNCH				
DINNER				
SNACKS				

HYDRATION

(8 cup icons)

SUPPLEMENTS

☺

HOURS SLEPT LAST NIGHT

Z Z Z Z Z Z Z +

EXERCISE

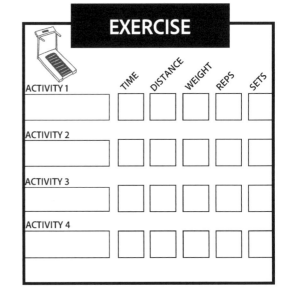

	TIME	DISTANCE	WEIGHT	REPS	SETS
ACTIVITY 1					
ACTIVITY 2					
ACTIVITY 3					
ACTIVITY 4					

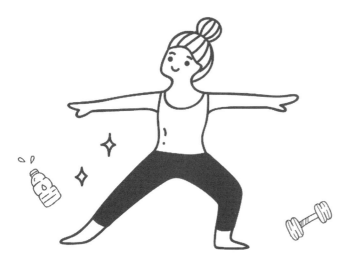

Mind & Spirit

PRAYER/MEDITATION 🙏

Reflections:

_____

_____

_____

SELF - CARE 🖤

I looked after me by:

_____

_____

_____

GRATITUDE ⭐

I am grateful for:

_____

_____

_____

TODAY I FEEL 😮 🙂 😢 😐 😠

_____

_____

Taking Care of Body.

DATE: _____   S M T W T F S

TODAY'S GOALS

MEALS

	CALORIES	FAT	PROTEIN	CARBS
BREAKFAST				
LUNCH				
DINNER				
SNACKS				

HYDRATION

SUPPLEMENTS

☺

HOURS SLEPT LAST NIGHT

Z Z Z Z Z Z Z +

EXERCISE

	TIME	DISTANCE	WEIGHT	REPS	SETS
ACTIVITY 1					
ACTIVITY 2					
ACTIVITY 3					
ACTIVITY 4					

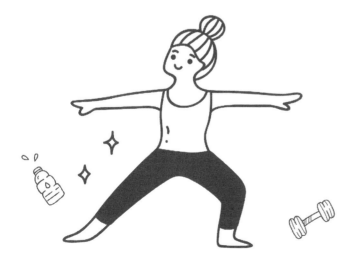

Mind & Spirit

PRAYER/MEDITATION 🙏

Reflections:

_____

_____

_____

SELF - CARE ♥

I looked after me by:

_____

_____

_____

GRATITUDE ⭐

I am grateful for:

_____

_____

_____

TODAY I FEEL 😲 🙂 😢 😐 😠

_____

_____

Taking Care of Body,

DATE: [   ]   S M T W T F S

TODAY'S GOALS

MEALS

	CALORIES	FAT	PROTEIN	CARBS
BREAKFAST				
LUNCH				
DINNER				
SNACKS				

HYDRATION

SUPPLEMENTS
☺

HOURS SLEPT LAST NIGHT
Z Z Z Z Z Z Z +

EXERCISE

	TIME	DISTANCE	WEIGHT	REPS	SETS
ACTIVITY 1					
ACTIVITY 2					
ACTIVITY 3					
ACTIVITY 4					

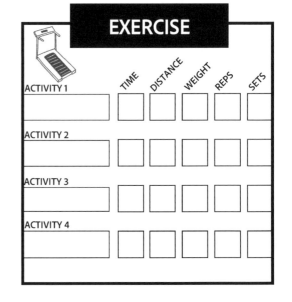

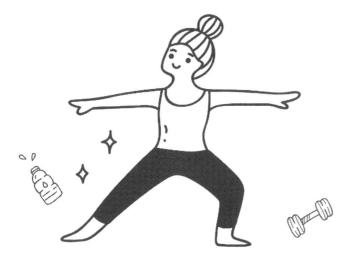

Mind & Spirit

PRAYER/MEDITATION 🙏

Reflections:

_____

_____

_____

SELF - CARE 🖤

I looked after me by:

_____

_____

_____

GRATITUDE ⭐

I am grateful for:

_____

_____

_____

TODAY I FEEL 😲 🙂 😢 😐 😠

_____

_____

Taking Care of Body,

TODAY'S GOALS

MEALS

	CALORIES	FAT	PROTEIN	CARBS
BREAKFAST				
LUNCH				
DINNER				
SNACKS				

HYDRATION

SUPPLEMENTS

☺

HOURS SLEPT LAST NIGHT

Z Z Z Z Z Z Z +

EXERCISE

	TIME	DISTANCE	WEIGHT	REPS	SETS
ACTIVITY 1					
ACTIVITY 2					
ACTIVITY 3					
ACTIVITY 4					

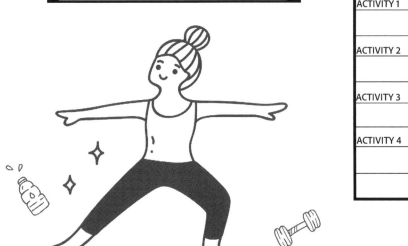

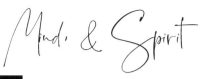

Mind & Spirit

PRAYER/MEDITATION 🙏

Reflections:

_____

_____

_____

SELF - CARE 🖤

I looked after me by:

_____

_____

_____

GRATITUDE ⭐

I am grateful for:

_____

_____

_____

TODAY I FEEL 😮 🙂 😢 😐 😠

_____

_____

Taking Care of Body.

DATE: _____   S M T W T F S

TODAY'S GOALS

MEALS

	CALORIES	FAT	PROTEIN	CARBS
BREAKFAST				
LUNCH				
DINNER				
SNACKS				

HYDRATION

SUPPLEMENTS

:)

HOURS SLEPT LAST NIGHT

Z Z Z Z Z Z Z +

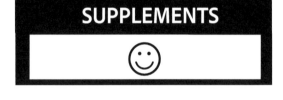

EXERCISE

	TIME	DISTANCE	WEIGHT	REPS	SETS
ACTIVITY 1					
ACTIVITY 2					
ACTIVITY 3					
ACTIVITY 4					

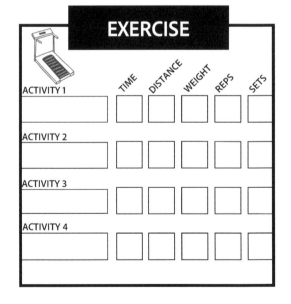

Mind & Spirit

PRAYER/MEDITATION 🙏

Reflections: _____
_____
_____
_____

SELF - CARE ♥

I looked after me by: _____
_____
_____
_____

GRATITUDE ⭐

I am grateful for: _____
_____
_____
_____

TODAY I FEEL 😮 🙂 😢 😐 😠

_____
_____

Taking Care of Body

DATE: _____

S M T W T F S

TODAY'S GOALS

MEALS

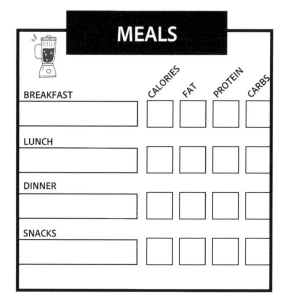

	CALORIES	FAT	PROTEIN	CARBS
BREAKFAST				
LUNCH				
DINNER				
SNACKS				

HYDRATION

SUPPLEMENTS

:)

HOURS SLEPT LAST NIGHT

Z Z Z Z Z Z Z +

EXERCISE

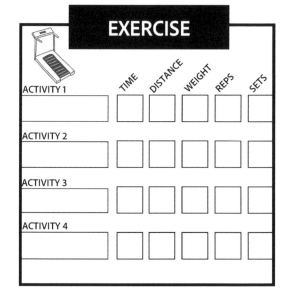

	TIME	DISTANCE	WEIGHT	REPS	SETS
ACTIVITY 1					
ACTIVITY 2					
ACTIVITY 3					
ACTIVITY 4					

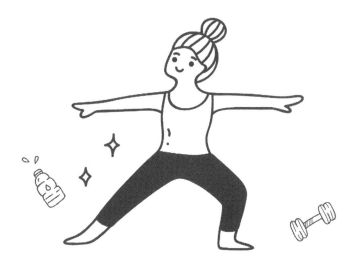

Mind & Spirit

PRAYER/MEDITATION 🙏

Reflections:

_____

_____

_____

_____

SELF - CARE 🖤

I looked after me by:

_____

_____

_____

GRATITUDE ⭐

I am grateful for:

_____

_____

_____

TODAY I FEEL 😮 🙂 😢 😐 😠

_____

_____

Taking Care of Body,

DATE: _____   S M T W T F S

TODAY'S GOALS

(blank lined list)

MEALS

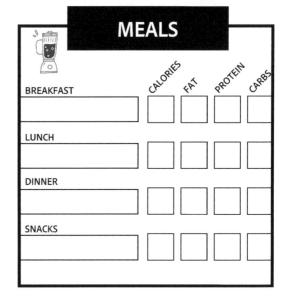

	CALORIES	FAT	PROTEIN	CARBS
BREAKFAST				
LUNCH				
DINNER				
SNACKS				

HYDRATION

(8 cup icons)

SUPPLEMENTS

☺

HOURS SLEPT LAST NIGHT

Z Z Z Z Z Z Z +

EXERCISE

	TIME	DISTANCE	WEIGHT	REPS	SETS
ACTIVITY 1					
ACTIVITY 2					
ACTIVITY 3					
ACTIVITY 4					

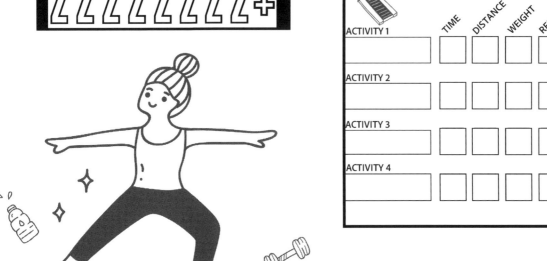

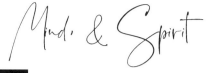

Mind & Spirit

PRAYER/MEDITATION 🙏

Reflections:

_____

_____

_____

SELF - CARE 🖤

I looked after me by:

_____

_____

_____

GRATITUDE ⭐

I am grateful for:

_____

_____

_____

TODAY I FEEL 😲 🙂 😢 😐 😠

_____

_____

Taking Care of Body,

DATE: [_____] S M T W T F S

TODAY'S GOALS

MEALS

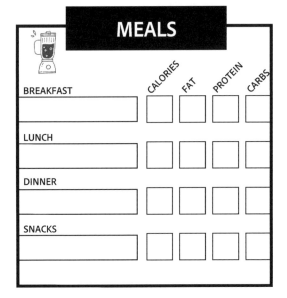

	CALORIES	FAT	PROTEIN	CARBS
BREAKFAST				
LUNCH				
DINNER				
SNACKS				

HYDRATION

SUPPLEMENTS

😊

HOURS SLEPT LAST NIGHT

Z Z Z Z Z Z Z +

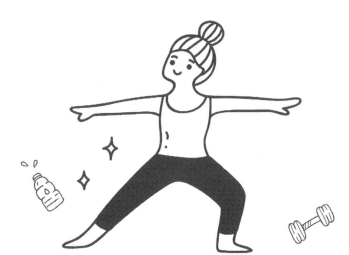

EXERCISE

	TIME	DISTANCE	WEIGHT	REPS	SETS
ACTIVITY 1					
ACTIVITY 2					
ACTIVITY 3					
ACTIVITY 4					

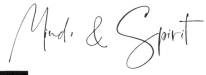

Mind & Spirit

PRAYER/MEDITATION 🙏

Reflections:

_____
_____
_____
_____

SELF - CARE 🖤

I looked after me by:

_____
_____
_____
_____

GRATITUDE ⭐

I am grateful for:

_____
_____
_____
_____

TODAY I FEEL 😲 🙂 😢 😐 😠

_____
_____

Taking Care of Body

DATE: [   ]   **S M T W T F S**

TODAY'S GOALS

MEALS

	CALORIES	FAT	PROTEIN	CARBS
BREAKFAST				
LUNCH				
DINNER				
SNACKS				

HYDRATION

SUPPLEMENTS

☺

HOURS SLEPT LAST NIGHT

Z Z Z Z Z Z Z +

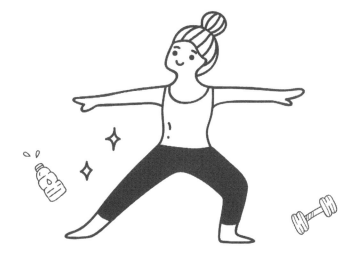

EXERCISE

	TIME	DISTANCE	WEIGHT	REPS	SETS
ACTIVITY 1					
ACTIVITY 2					
ACTIVITY 3					
ACTIVITY 4					

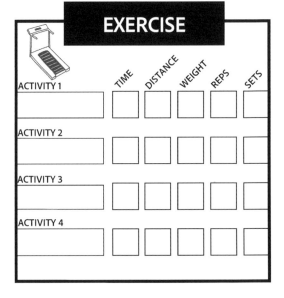

Mind & Spirit

PRAYER/MEDITATION 🙏

Reflections:

_____
_____
_____
_____

SELF - CARE 🖤

I looked after me by:

_____
_____
_____
_____

GRATITUDE ⭐

I am grateful for:

_____
_____
_____
_____

TODAY I FEEL 😮 🙂 😢 😐 😠

_____
_____

Taking Care of Body,

DATE: _____   S M T W T F S

TODAY'S GOALS

MEALS

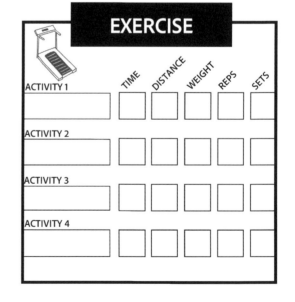

	CALORIES	FAT	PROTEIN	CARBS
BREAKFAST				
LUNCH				
DINNER				
SNACKS				

HYDRATION

SUPPLEMENTS

☺

HOURS SLEPT LAST NIGHT

Z Z Z Z Z Z Z +

EXERCISE

	TIME	DISTANCE	WEIGHT	REPS	SETS
ACTIVITY 1					
ACTIVITY 2					
ACTIVITY 3					
ACTIVITY 4					

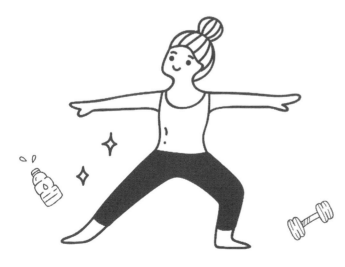

Mind & Spirit

PRAYER/MEDITATION 🙏

Reflections:

_____

_____

_____

_____

SELF - CARE 🖤

I looked after me by:

_____

_____

_____

_____

GRATITUDE ⭐

I am grateful for:

_____

_____

_____

_____

TODAY I FEEL 😲 🙂 😢 😐 😠

_____

_____

Taking Care of Body

DATE: _____   S M T W T F S

TODAY'S GOALS

MEALS

	CALORIES	FAT	PROTEIN	CARBS
BREAKFAST				
LUNCH				
DINNER				
SNACKS				

HYDRATION

SUPPLEMENTS

☺

HOURS SLEPT LAST NIGHT

Z Z Z Z Z Z Z +

EXERCISE

	TIME	DISTANCE	WEIGHT	REPS	SETS
ACTIVITY 1					
ACTIVITY 2					
ACTIVITY 3					
ACTIVITY 4					

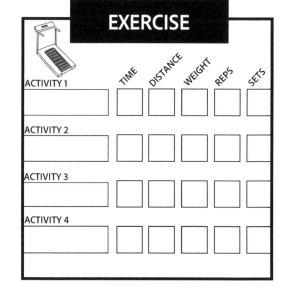

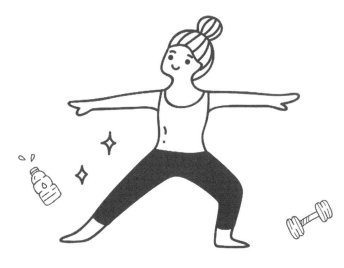

Mind & Spirit

PRAYER/MEDITATION 🙏

Reflections:

_____

_____

_____

SELF - CARE 🖤

I looked after me by:

_____

_____

_____

GRATITUDE ⭐

I am grateful for:

_____

_____

_____

TODAY I FEEL 😮 🙂 😢 😐 😠

_____

_____

Taking Care of Body.

DATE: _____   S M T W T F S

TODAY'S GOALS

MEALS

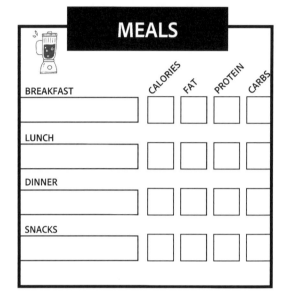

	CALORIES	FAT	PROTEIN	CARBS
BREAKFAST				
LUNCH				
DINNER				
SNACKS				

HYDRATION

SUPPLEMENTS

☺

HOURS SLEPT LAST NIGHT

Z Z Z Z Z Z Z +

EXERCISE

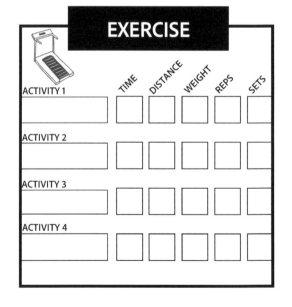

	TIME	DISTANCE	WEIGHT	REPS	SETS
ACTIVITY 1					
ACTIVITY 2					
ACTIVITY 3					
ACTIVITY 4					

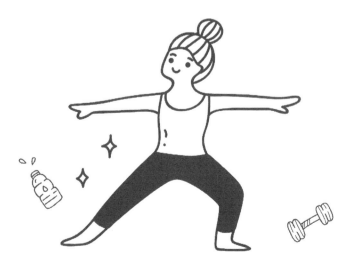

Mind & Spirit

PRAYER/MEDITATION 🙏

Reflections:

_____

_____

_____

SELF - CARE 🖤

I looked after me by:

_____

_____

_____

GRATITUDE ⭐

I am grateful for:

_____

_____

_____

TODAY I FEEL 😮 🙂 😢 😐 😠

_____

_____

Taking Care of Body,

DATE: _____   S M T W T F S

TODAY'S GOALS

(blank lined list)

MEALS

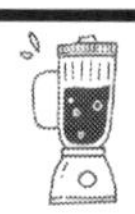

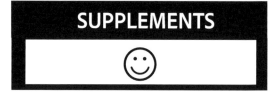

	CALORIES	FAT	PROTEIN	CARBS
BREAKFAST				
LUNCH				
DINNER				
SNACKS				

HYDRATION

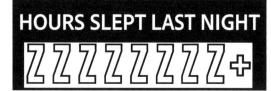

SUPPLEMENTS

☺

HOURS SLEPT LAST NIGHT

Z Z Z Z Z Z Z +

EXERCISE

	TIME	DISTANCE	WEIGHT	REPS	SETS
ACTIVITY 1					
ACTIVITY 2					
ACTIVITY 3					
ACTIVITY 4					

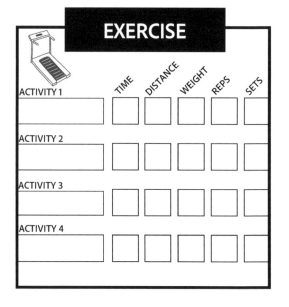

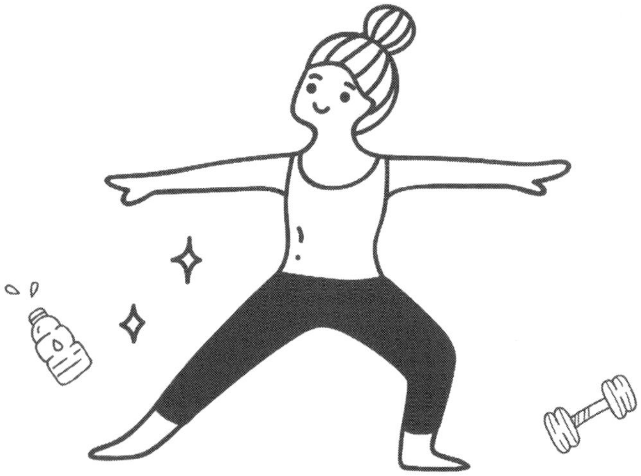

Mind & Spirit

PRAYER/MEDITATION 🙏

Reflections:

_____

_____

_____

SELF - CARE 🖤

I looked after me by:

_____

_____

_____

GRATITUDE ⭐

I am grateful for:

_____

_____

_____

TODAY I FEEL 😲 🙂 🥲 😐 😠

_____

_____

Taking Care of Body,

DATE: _____   S M T W T F S

TODAY'S GOALS

MEALS

	CALORIES	FAT	PROTEIN	CARBS
BREAKFAST				
LUNCH				
DINNER				
SNACKS				

HYDRATION

SUPPLEMENTS

☺

HOURS SLEPT LAST NIGHT

Z Z Z Z Z Z Z +

EXERCISE

	TIME	DISTANCE	WEIGHT	REPS	SETS
ACTIVITY 1					
ACTIVITY 2					
ACTIVITY 3					
ACTIVITY 4					

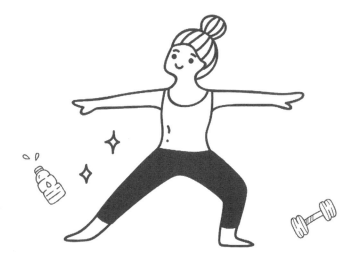

Mind & Spirit

PRAYER/MEDITATION 🙏

Reflections:

_____
_____
_____

SELF - CARE 🖤

I looked after me by:

_____
_____
_____

GRATITUDE ⭐

I am grateful for:

_____
_____
_____

TODAY I FEEL 😲 🙂 😢 😐 😠

_____
_____

Taking Care of Body

DATE: _____   S M T W T F S

TODAY'S GOALS

MEALS

	CALORIES	FAT	PROTEIN	CARBS
BREAKFAST				
LUNCH				
DINNER				
SNACKS				

HYDRATION

SUPPLEMENTS

☺

HOURS SLEPT LAST NIGHT

Z Z Z Z Z Z Z +

EXERCISE

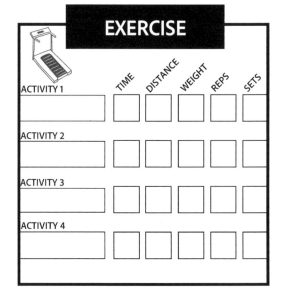

	TIME	DISTANCE	WEIGHT	REPS	SETS
ACTIVITY 1					
ACTIVITY 2					
ACTIVITY 3					
ACTIVITY 4					

Mind & Spirit

PRAYER/MEDITATION

Reflections:

_____
_____
_____
_____

SELF - CARE ♥

I looked after me by:

_____
_____
_____
_____

GRATITUDE ⭐

I am grateful for:

_____
_____
_____
_____

TODAY I FEEL 😮 🙂 😢 😐 😠

_____
_____

Taking Care of Body.

DATE: _____ S M T W T F S

TODAY'S GOALS

MEALS

	CALORIES	FAT	PROTEIN	CARBS
BREAKFAST				
LUNCH				
DINNER				
SNACKS				

HYDRATION

SUPPLEMENTS
☺

HOURS SLEPT LAST NIGHT
Z Z Z Z Z Z Z +

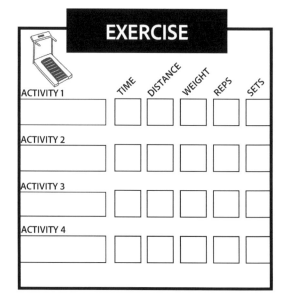

EXERCISE

	TIME	DISTANCE	WEIGHT	REPS	SETS
ACTIVITY 1					
ACTIVITY 2					
ACTIVITY 3					
ACTIVITY 4					

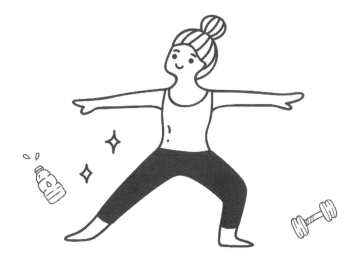

Mind, & Spirit

PRAYER/MEDITATION 🙏

Reflections:

_____

_____
_____
_____

SELF - CARE 🖤

I looked after me by:

_____

_____
_____
_____

GRATITUDE ⭐

I am grateful for:

_____

_____
_____
_____

TODAY I FEEL 😮 🙂 😢 😐 😠

_____

_____

Taking Care of Body.

DATE: _____   S M T W T F S

TODAY'S GOALS

MEALS

	CALORIES	FAT	PROTEIN	CARBS
BREAKFAST				
LUNCH				
DINNER				
SNACKS				

HYDRATION

SUPPLEMENTS

:)

HOURS SLEPT LAST NIGHT

Z Z Z Z Z Z Z +

EXERCISE

	TIME	DISTANCE	WEIGHT	REPS	SETS
ACTIVITY 1					
ACTIVITY 2					
ACTIVITY 3					
ACTIVITY 4					

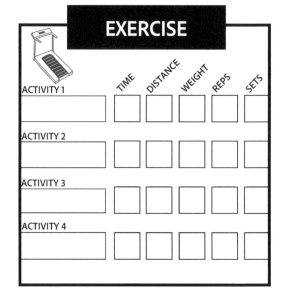

Mind & Spirit

PRAYER/MEDITATION 🙏

Reflections:

_____

_____

_____

_____

SELF - CARE 🖤

I looked after me by:

_____

_____

_____

_____

GRATITUDE ⭐

I am grateful for:

_____

_____

_____

_____

TODAY I FEEL 😮 🙂 😢 😐 😠

_____

_____

Taking Care of Body.

DATE: _____   **S M T W T F S**

TODAY'S GOALS

MEALS

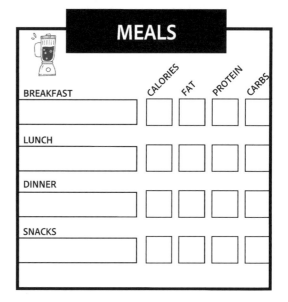

	CALORIES	FAT	PROTEIN	CARBS
BREAKFAST				
LUNCH				
DINNER				
SNACKS				

HYDRATION

SUPPLEMENTS

☺

HOURS SLEPT LAST NIGHT

Z Z Z Z Z Z Z +

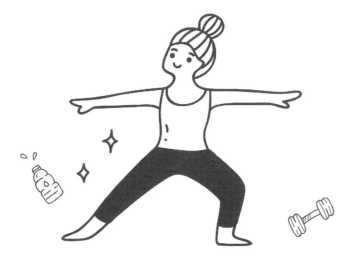

EXERCISE

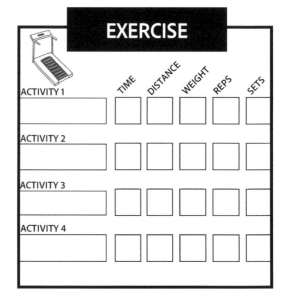

	TIME	DISTANCE	WEIGHT	REPS	SETS
ACTIVITY 1					
ACTIVITY 2					
ACTIVITY 3					
ACTIVITY 4					

Mind & Spirit

PRAYER/MEDITATION 🙏

Reflections:

_____

_____

_____

SELF - CARE 🖤

I looked after me by:

_____

_____

_____

GRATITUDE ⭐

I am grateful for:

_____

_____

_____

TODAY I FEEL 😮 🙂 😢 😐 😠

_____

_____

Taking Care of Body,

DATE: [_____] | S M T W T F S

TODAY'S GOALS

MEALS

	CALORIES	FAT	PROTEIN	CARBS
BREAKFAST				
LUNCH				
DINNER				
SNACKS				

HYDRATION

SUPPLEMENTS

☺

HOURS SLEPT LAST NIGHT

Z Z Z Z Z Z Z +

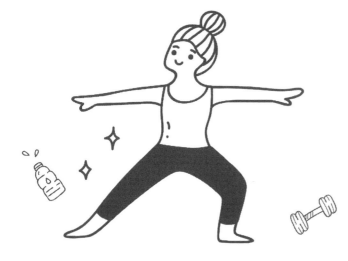

EXERCISE

	TIME	DISTANCE	WEIGHT	REPS	SETS
ACTIVITY 1					
ACTIVITY 2					
ACTIVITY 3					
ACTIVITY 4					

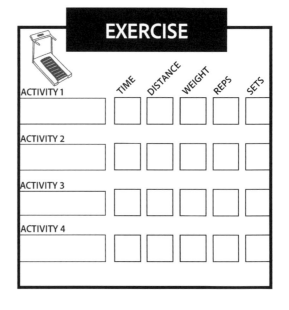

Mind & Spirit

PRAYER/MEDITATION 🙏

Reflections:

_____
_____
_____

SELF - CARE 🖤

I looked after me by:

_____
_____
_____

GRATITUDE ⭐

I am grateful for:

_____
_____
_____

TODAY I FEEL 😲 🙂 😢 😐 😠

_____
_____

Taking Care of Body,

DATE: [   ]   S M T W T F S

TODAY'S GOALS

MEALS

	CALORIES	FAT	PROTEIN	CARBS
BREAKFAST				
LUNCH				
DINNER				
SNACKS				

HYDRATION

SUPPLEMENTS

:)

HOURS SLEPT LAST NIGHT

Z Z Z Z Z Z Z +

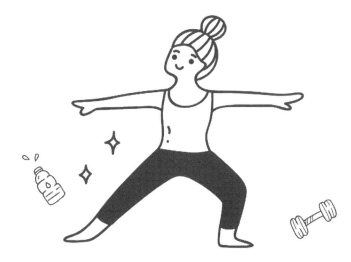

EXERCISE

	TIME	DISTANCE	WEIGHT	REPS	SETS
ACTIVITY 1					
ACTIVITY 2					
ACTIVITY 3					
ACTIVITY 4					

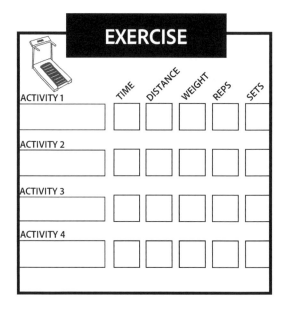

Mind & Spirit

PRAYER/MEDITATION 🙏

Reflections:

_____

_____

_____

SELF - CARE 🖤

I looked after me by:

_____

_____

_____

GRATITUDE ⭐

I am grateful for:

_____

_____

_____

TODAY I FEEL 😮 🙂 🥲 😐 😠

_____

_____

Taking Care of Body

DATE: _____   S M T W T F S

TODAY'S GOALS

MEALS

	CALORIES	FAT	PROTEIN	CARBS
BREAKFAST				
LUNCH				
DINNER				
SNACKS				

HYDRATION

SUPPLEMENTS

🙂

HOURS SLEPT LAST NIGHT

Z Z Z Z Z Z Z +

EXERCISE

	TIME	DISTANCE	WEIGHT	REPS	SETS
ACTIVITY 1					
ACTIVITY 2					
ACTIVITY 3					
ACTIVITY 4					

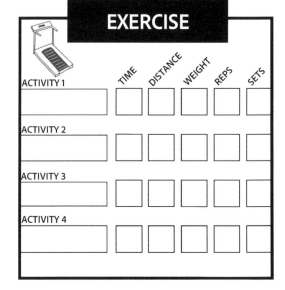
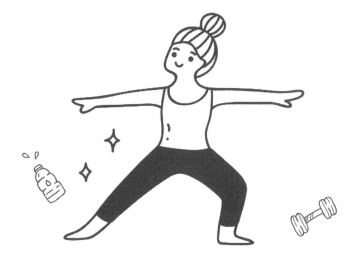

Mind & Spirit

PRAYER/MEDITATION 🙏

Reflections:

_____

_____

_____

SELF - CARE ♥

I looked after me by:

_____

_____

_____

GRATITUDE ⭐

I am grateful for:

_____

_____

_____

TODAY I FEEL 😲 🙂 😢 😐 😠

_____

_____

Taking Care of Body,

DATE: _____ S M T W T F S

TODAY'S GOALS

MEALS

	CALORIES	FAT	PROTEIN	CARBS
BREAKFAST				
LUNCH				
DINNER				
SNACKS				

HYDRATION

SUPPLEMENTS

☺

HOURS SLEPT LAST NIGHT

Z Z Z Z Z Z Z +

EXERCISE

	TIME	DISTANCE	WEIGHT	REPS	SETS
ACTIVITY 1					
ACTIVITY 2					
ACTIVITY 3					
ACTIVITY 4					

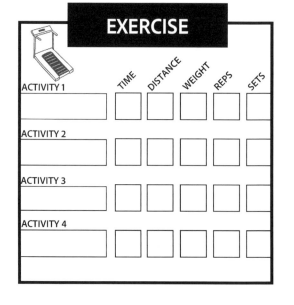

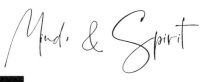

PRAYER/MEDITATION 🙏

Reflections:

_____
_____
_____

SELF - CARE 🖤

I looked after me by:

_____
_____
_____

GRATITUDE ⭐

I am grateful for:

_____
_____
_____

TODAY I FEEL 😮 🙂 😢 😐 😠

_____
_____

Taking Care of Body,

DATE: [   ]   S M T W T F S

TODAY'S GOALS

MEALS

	CALORIES	FAT	PROTEIN	CARBS
BREAKFAST				
LUNCH				
DINNER				
SNACKS				

HYDRATION

SUPPLEMENTS

☺

HOURS SLEPT LAST NIGHT

Z Z Z Z Z Z Z +

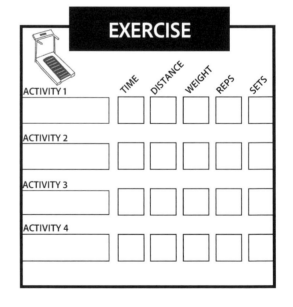

EXERCISE

	TIME	DISTANCE	WEIGHT	REPS	SETS
ACTIVITY 1					
ACTIVITY 2					
ACTIVITY 3					
ACTIVITY 4					

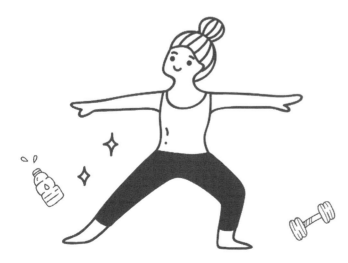

Mind & Spirit

PRAYER/MEDITATION 🙏

Reflections:

_____
_____
_____

SELF - CARE 🖤

I looked after me by:

_____
_____
_____

GRATITUDE ⭐

I am grateful for:

_____
_____
_____

TODAY I FEEL 😮 🙂 🥺 😐 😠

_____
_____

Taking Care of Body,

DATE: [_____]   S M T W T F S

TODAY'S GOALS

MEALS

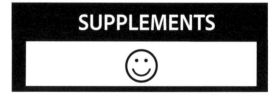

	CALORIES	FAT	PROTEIN	CARBS
BREAKFAST				
LUNCH				
DINNER				
SNACKS				

HYDRATION

SUPPLEMENTS

☺

HOURS SLEPT LAST NIGHT

Z Z Z Z Z Z Z +

EXERCISE

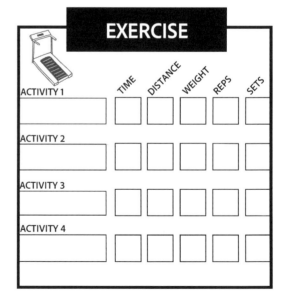

	TIME	DISTANCE	WEIGHT	REPS	SETS
ACTIVITY 1					
ACTIVITY 2					
ACTIVITY 3					
ACTIVITY 4					

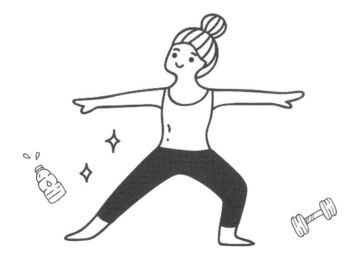

Mind & Spirit

PRAYER/MEDITATION 🙏

Reflections:

_____

_____

_____

_____

SELF - CARE 💜

I looked after me by:

_____

_____

_____

_____

GRATITUDE ⭐

I am grateful for:

_____

_____

_____

_____

TODAY I FEEL 😮 🙂 😢 😐 😠

_____

_____

Taking Care of Body

DATE: _____

S M T W T F S

TODAY'S GOALS

MEALS

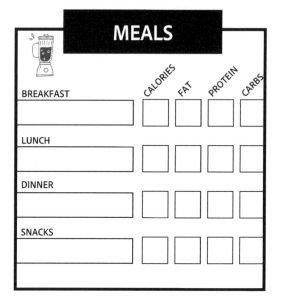

	CALORIES	FAT	PROTEIN	CARBS
BREAKFAST				
LUNCH				
DINNER				
SNACKS				

HYDRATION

SUPPLEMENTS

☺

HOURS SLEPT LAST NIGHT

Z Z Z Z Z Z Z +

EXERCISE

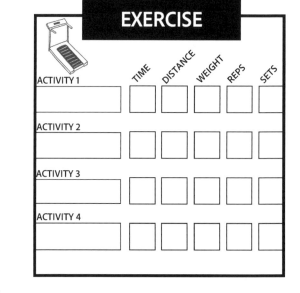

	TIME	DISTANCE	WEIGHT	REPS	SETS
ACTIVITY 1					
ACTIVITY 2					
ACTIVITY 3					
ACTIVITY 4					

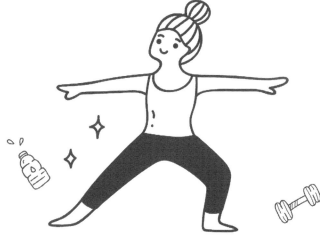

Mind & Spirit

PRAYER/MEDITATION 🙏

Reflections:

_____

_____

_____

SELF - CARE ♥

I looked after me by:

_____

_____

_____

GRATITUDE ⭐

I am grateful for:

_____

_____

_____

TODAY I FEEL 😮 🙂 😢 😐 😠

_____

_____

Taking Care of Body.

DATE: _____   S M T W T F S

TODAY'S GOALS

(blank lined list)

MEALS

	CALORIES	FAT	PROTEIN	CARBS
BREAKFAST				
LUNCH				
DINNER				
SNACKS				

HYDRATION

(eight cup icons)

SUPPLEMENTS

☺

HOURS SLEPT LAST NIGHT

Z Z Z Z Z Z Z +

EXERCISE

	TIME	DISTANCE	WEIGHT	REPS	SETS
ACTIVITY 1					
ACTIVITY 2					
ACTIVITY 3					
ACTIVITY 4					

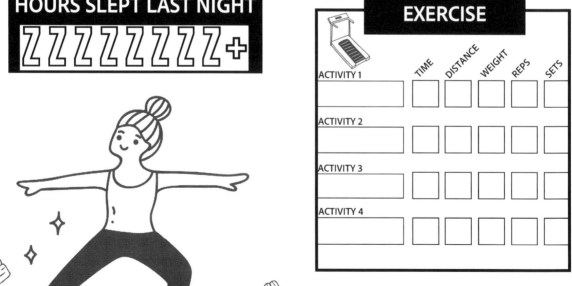

Mind & Spirit

PRAYER/MEDITATION 🙏

Reflections:

_____
_____
_____

SELF - CARE ♥

I looked after me by:

_____
_____
_____

GRATITUDE ⭐

I am grateful for:

_____
_____
_____

TODAY I FEEL 😲 🙂 😢 😐 😠

_____
_____

Taking Care of Body,

DATE: _____   S M T W T F S

TODAY'S GOALS

MEALS

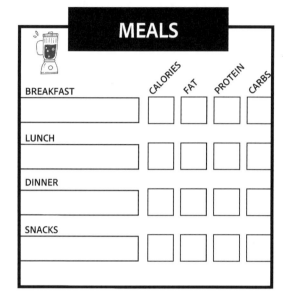

	CALORIES	FAT	PROTEIN	CARBS
BREAKFAST				
LUNCH				
DINNER				
SNACKS				

HYDRATION

SUPPLEMENTS

☺

HOURS SLEPT LAST NIGHT

Z Z Z Z Z Z Z +

EXERCISE

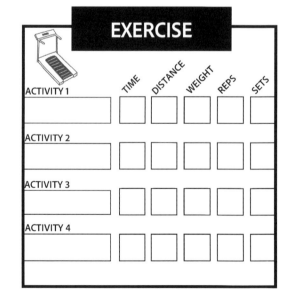

	TIME	DISTANCE	WEIGHT	REPS	SETS
ACTIVITY 1					
ACTIVITY 2					
ACTIVITY 3					
ACTIVITY 4					

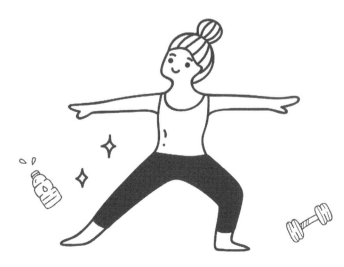

Mind & Spirit

PRAYER/MEDITATION 🙏

Reflections:

_____

_____

_____

SELF - CARE 🖤

I looked after me by:

_____

_____

_____

GRATITUDE ⭐

I am grateful for:

_____

_____

_____

TODAY I FEEL 😮 🙂 😢 😐 😠

_____

_____

Taking Care of Body

DATE: _____   S M T W T F S

TODAY'S GOALS

MEALS

	CALORIES	FAT	PROTEIN	CARBS
BREAKFAST				
LUNCH				
DINNER				
SNACKS				

HYDRATION

SUPPLEMENTS

HOURS SLEPT LAST NIGHT

Z Z Z Z Z Z Z +

EXERCISE

	TIME	DISTANCE	WEIGHT	REPS	SETS
ACTIVITY 1					
ACTIVITY 2					
ACTIVITY 3					
ACTIVITY 4					

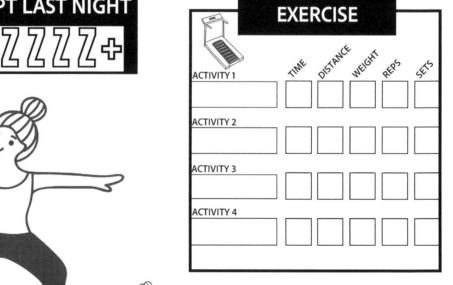

Mind & Spirit

PRAYER/MEDITATION 🙏

Reflections:

_____

_____

_____

SELF - CARE 🖤

I looked after me by:

_____

_____

_____

GRATITUDE ⭐

I am grateful for:

_____

_____

_____

TODAY I FEEL 😮 🙂 😢 😐 😠

_____

_____

Taking Care of Body

DATE: _____   S M T W T F S

TODAY'S GOALS

MEALS

	CALORIES	FAT	PROTEIN	CARBS
BREAKFAST				
LUNCH				
DINNER				
SNACKS				

HYDRATION

SUPPLEMENTS

:)

HOURS SLEPT LAST NIGHT

Z Z Z Z Z Z Z +

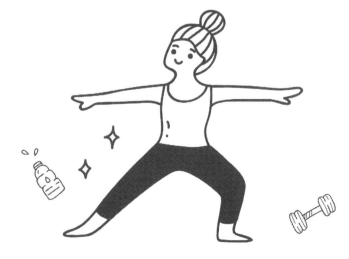

EXERCISE

	TIME	DISTANCE	WEIGHT	REPS	SETS
ACTIVITY 1					
ACTIVITY 2					
ACTIVITY 3					
ACTIVITY 4					

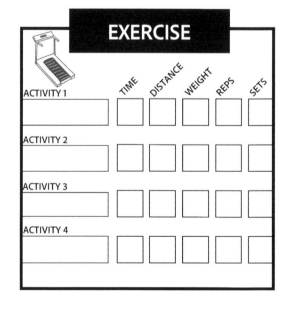

Mind & Spirit

PRAYER/MEDITATION 🙏

Reflections:

_____

_____

_____

SELF - CARE 🖤

I looked after me by:

_____

_____

_____

GRATITUDE ⭐

I am grateful for:

_____

_____

_____

TODAY I FEEL 😲 🙂 😢 😐 😠

_____

_____

Taking Care of Body,

TODAY'S GOALS

MEALS

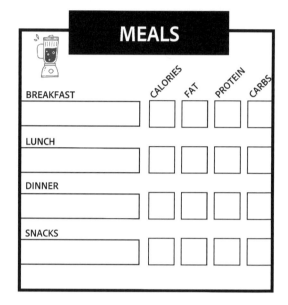

	CALORIES	FAT	PROTEIN	CARBS
BREAKFAST				
LUNCH				
DINNER				
SNACKS				

HYDRATION

SUPPLEMENTS

☺

HOURS SLEPT LAST NIGHT

Z Z Z Z Z Z Z ✚

EXERCISE

	TIME	DISTANCE	WEIGHT	REPS	SETS
ACTIVITY 1					
ACTIVITY 2					
ACTIVITY 3					
ACTIVITY 4					

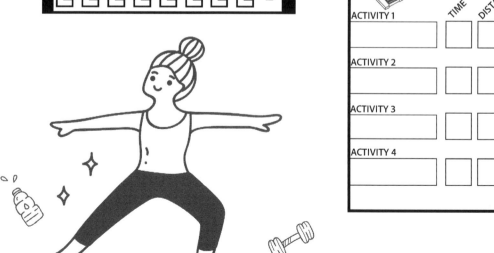

Mind & Spirit

PRAYER/MEDITATION 🙏

Reflections:

_____

_____

_____

SELF - CARE 🖤

I looked after me by:

_____

_____

_____

GRATITUDE ⭐

I am grateful for:

_____

_____

_____

TODAY I FEEL 😮 🙂 😢 😐 😠

_____

_____

Taking Care of Body,

DATE: _____   S M T W T F S

TODAY'S GOALS

_____
_____
_____
_____
_____
_____
_____
_____

MEALS

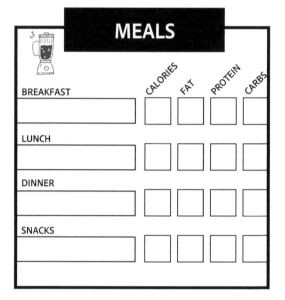

	CALORIES	FAT	PROTEIN	CARBS
BREAKFAST				
LUNCH				
DINNER				
SNACKS				

HYDRATION

SUPPLEMENTS

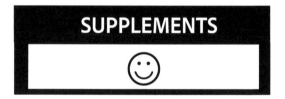

HOURS SLEPT LAST NIGHT

Z Z Z Z Z Z Z +

EXERCISE

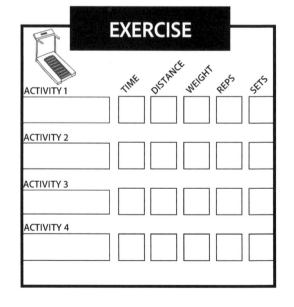

	TIME	DISTANCE	WEIGHT	REPS	SETS
ACTIVITY 1					
ACTIVITY 2					
ACTIVITY 3					
ACTIVITY 4					

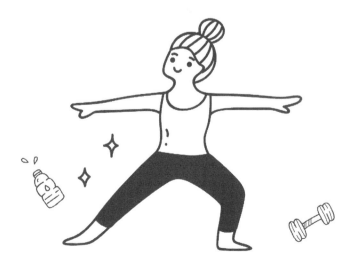

Mind & Spirit

PRAYER/MEDITATION 🙏

Reflections:

_____

_____

_____

SELF - CARE 🖤

I looked after me by:

_____

_____

_____

GRATITUDE ⭐

I am grateful for:

_____

_____

_____

TODAY I FEEL 😲 🙂 😢 😐 😠

_____

_____

Taking Care of Body,

DATE: _____   **S M T W T F S**

TODAY'S GOALS

MEALS

	CALORIES	FAT	PROTEIN	CARBS
BREAKFAST				
LUNCH				
DINNER				
SNACKS				

HYDRATION

SUPPLEMENTS

☺

HOURS SLEPT LAST NIGHT

Z Z Z Z Z Z Z ✚

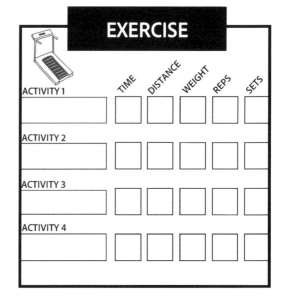

EXERCISE

	TIME	DISTANCE	WEIGHT	REPS	SETS
ACTIVITY 1					
ACTIVITY 2					
ACTIVITY 3					
ACTIVITY 4					

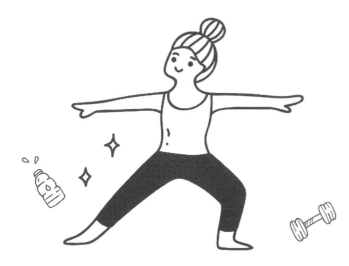

Mind & Spirit

PRAYER/MEDITATION 🙏

Reflections:

_____

_____

_____

_____

SELF - CARE 🖤

I looked after me by:

_____

_____

_____

_____

GRATITUDE ⭐

I am grateful for:

_____

_____

_____

_____

TODAY I FEEL 😮 🙂 😢 😐 😠

_____

_____

Taking Care of Body,

DATE: _____   S M T W T F S

TODAY'S GOALS

MEALS

	CALORIES	FAT	PROTEIN	CARBS
BREAKFAST				
LUNCH				
DINNER				
SNACKS				

HYDRATION

SUPPLEMENTS

☺

HOURS SLEPT LAST NIGHT

Z Z Z Z Z Z Z ✚

EXERCISE

	TIME	DISTANCE	WEIGHT	REPS	SETS
ACTIVITY 1					
ACTIVITY 2					
ACTIVITY 3					
ACTIVITY 4					

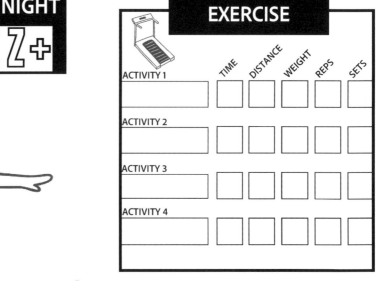

Mind & Spirit

PRAYER/MEDITATION 🙏

Reflections:

_____
_____
_____
_____

SELF - CARE 🖤

I looked after me by:

_____
_____
_____
_____

GRATITUDE ⭐

I am grateful for:

_____
_____
_____
_____

TODAY I FEEL 😲 🙂 😢 😐 😠

_____
_____

Taking Care of Body.

TODAY'S GOALS

MEALS

	CALORIES	FAT	PROTEIN	CARBS
BREAKFAST				
LUNCH				
DINNER				
SNACKS				

HYDRATION

SUPPLEMENTS

☺

HOURS SLEPT LAST NIGHT

Z Z Z Z Z Z Z +

EXERCISE

	TIME	DISTANCE	WEIGHT	REPS	SETS
ACTIVITY 1					
ACTIVITY 2					
ACTIVITY 3					
ACTIVITY 4					

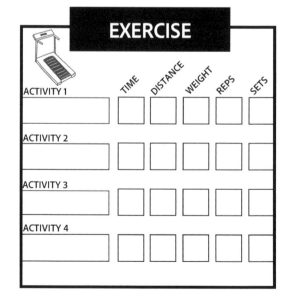

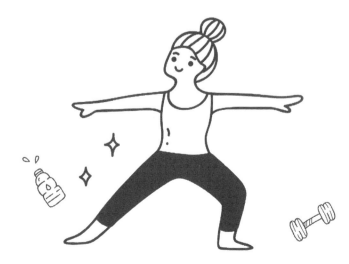

Mind & Spirit

PRAYER/MEDITATION 🙏

Reflections:

_____

_____

_____

SELF - CARE 💜

I looked after me by:

_____

_____

_____

GRATITUDE ⭐

I am grateful for:

_____

_____

_____

TODAY I FEEL 😲 🙂 😢 😐 😠

_____

_____

Taking Care of Body.

DATE: ⬜   **S M T W T F S**

TODAY'S GOALS

MEALS

	CALORIES	FAT	PROTEIN	CARBS
BREAKFAST				
LUNCH				
DINNER				
SNACKS				

HYDRATION

SUPPLEMENTS

🙂

HOURS SLEPT LAST NIGHT

Z Z Z Z Z Z Z +

EXERCISE

	TIME	DISTANCE	WEIGHT	REPS	SETS
ACTIVITY 1					
ACTIVITY 2					
ACTIVITY 3					
ACTIVITY 4					

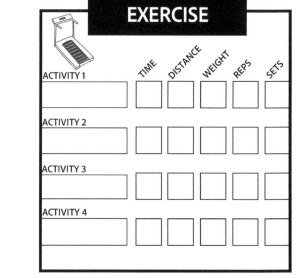

Mind & Spirit

PRAYER/MEDITATION 🙏

Reflections:

_____

_____

_____

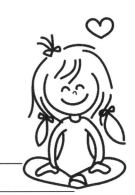

SELF - CARE 🖤

I looked after me by:

_____

_____

_____

GRATITUDE ⭐

I am grateful for:

_____

_____

_____

TODAY I FEEL 😲 🙂 😢 😐 😠

_____

_____

Taking Care of Body.

DATE: _____   S M T W T F S

TODAY'S GOALS

MEALS

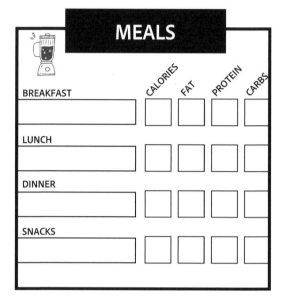

	CALORIES	FAT	PROTEIN	CARBS
BREAKFAST				
LUNCH				
DINNER				
SNACKS				

HYDRATION

🥤 🥤 🥤 🥤 🥤 🥤 🥤 🥤

SUPPLEMENTS

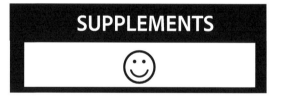

🙂

HOURS SLEPT LAST NIGHT

Z Z Z Z Z Z Z +

EXERCISE

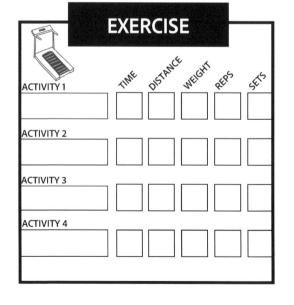

	TIME	DISTANCE	WEIGHT	REPS	SETS
ACTIVITY 1					
ACTIVITY 2					
ACTIVITY 3					
ACTIVITY 4					

Mind & Spirit

PRAYER/MEDITATION

Reflections:

_____
_____
_____
_____

SELF - CARE

I looked after me by:

_____
_____
_____
_____

GRATITUDE

I am grateful for:

_____
_____
_____
_____

TODAY I FEEL

_____
_____

Taking Care of Body

DATE: _____   S M T W T F S

TODAY'S GOALS

_____
_____
_____
_____
_____
_____
_____
_____
_____

MEALS

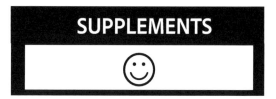

	CALORIES	FAT	PROTEIN	CARBS
BREAKFAST				
LUNCH				
DINNER				
SNACKS				

HYDRATION

SUPPLEMENTS

☺

HOURS SLEPT LAST NIGHT

Z Z Z Z Z Z Z ✚

EXERCISE

	TIME	DISTANCE	WEIGHT	REPS	SETS
ACTIVITY 1					
ACTIVITY 2					
ACTIVITY 3					
ACTIVITY 4					

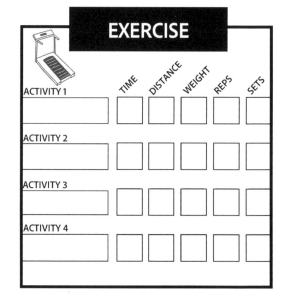

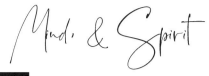

Mind & Spirit

PRAYER/MEDITATION

Reflections:

_____

_____

_____

SELF - CARE

I looked after me by:

_____

_____

_____

GRATITUDE

I am grateful for:

_____

_____

_____

TODAY I FEEL

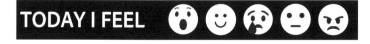

_____

_____

Taking Care of Body.

DATE: _____   **S M T W T F S**

TODAY'S GOALS

MEALS

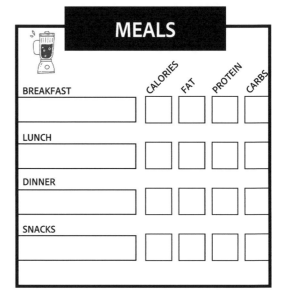

	CALORIES	FAT	PROTEIN	CARBS
BREAKFAST				
LUNCH				
DINNER				
SNACKS				

HYDRATION

SUPPLEMENTS

☺

HOURS SLEPT LAST NIGHT

Z Z Z Z Z Z Z +

EXERCISE

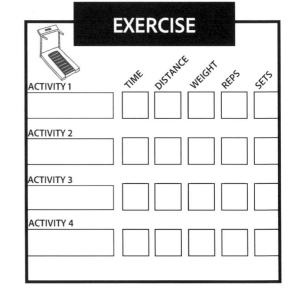

	TIME	DISTANCE	WEIGHT	REPS	SETS
ACTIVITY 1					
ACTIVITY 2					
ACTIVITY 3					
ACTIVITY 4					

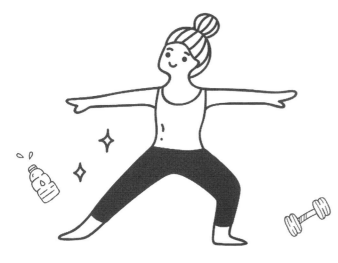

Mind & Spirit

PRAYER/MEDITATION 🙏

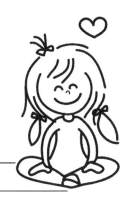

Reflections:

_____
_____
_____

SELF - CARE 🖤

I looked after me by:

_____
_____
_____

GRATITUDE ⭐

I am grateful for:

_____
_____
_____

TODAY I FEEL 😲 🙂 😢 😐 😠

_____
_____

Taking Care of Body.

DATE: [   ]   S M T W T F S

TODAY'S GOALS

MEALS

	CALORIES	FAT	PROTEIN	CARBS
BREAKFAST				
LUNCH				
DINNER				
SNACKS				

HYDRATION

SUPPLEMENTS

:)

HOURS SLEPT LAST NIGHT

Z Z Z Z Z Z Z +

EXERCISE

	TIME	DISTANCE	WEIGHT	REPS	SETS
ACTIVITY 1					
ACTIVITY 2					
ACTIVITY 3					
ACTIVITY 4					

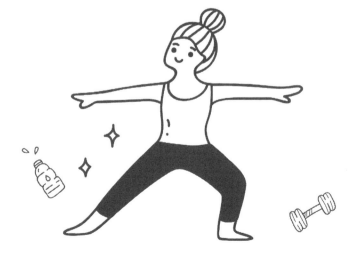

Mind & Spirit

PRAYER/MEDITATION 🙏

Reflections:

_____

_____

_____

SELF - CARE 🖤

I looked after me by:

_____

_____

_____

GRATITUDE ⭐

I am grateful for:

_____

_____

_____

TODAY I FEEL 😲 🙂 😢 😐 😠

_____

_____

Taking Care of Body,

DATE: [   ]   S M T W T F S

TODAY'S GOALS

MEALS

	CALORIES	FAT	PROTEIN	CARBS
BREAKFAST				
LUNCH				
DINNER				
SNACKS				

HYDRATION

SUPPLEMENTS

☺

HOURS SLEPT LAST NIGHT

Z Z Z Z Z Z Z +

EXERCISE

	TIME	DISTANCE	WEIGHT	REPS	SETS
ACTIVITY 1					
ACTIVITY 2					
ACTIVITY 3					
ACTIVITY 4					

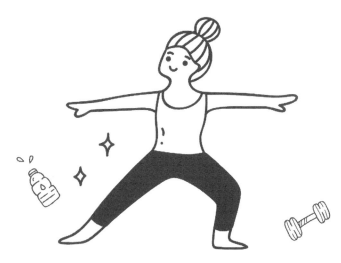
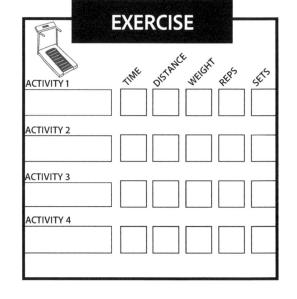

Mind. & Spirit

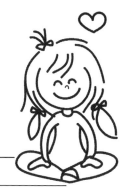

PRAYER/MEDITATION 🙏

Reflections:

_____

_____

_____

_____

SELF - CARE 🖤

I looked after me by:

_____

_____

_____

_____

GRATITUDE ⭐

I am grateful for:

_____

_____

_____

_____

TODAY I FEEL 😮 🙂 🥲 😐 😠

_____

_____

Taking Care of Body,

DATE: _____   S M T W T F S

TODAY'S GOALS

MEALS

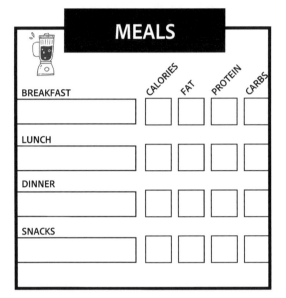

	CALORIES	FAT	PROTEIN	CARBS
BREAKFAST				
LUNCH				
DINNER				
SNACKS				

HYDRATION

SUPPLEMENTS

☺

HOURS SLEPT LAST NIGHT

Z Z Z Z Z Z Z +

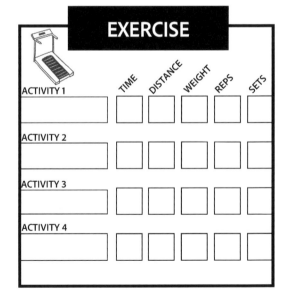

EXERCISE

	TIME	DISTANCE	WEIGHT	REPS	SETS
ACTIVITY 1					
ACTIVITY 2					
ACTIVITY 3					
ACTIVITY 4					

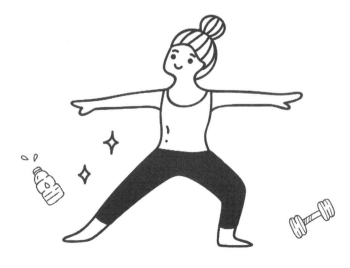

Mind & Spirit

PRAYER/MEDITATION 🙏

Reflections:

_____
_____
_____

SELF - CARE 💙

I looked after me by:

_____
_____
_____

GRATITUDE ⭐

I am grateful for:

_____
_____
_____

TODAY I FEEL 😲 🙂 😢 😐 😠

_____
_____

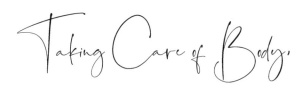

Taking Care of Body,

DATE: [   ]   S M T W T F S

TODAY'S GOALS

MEALS

	CALORIES	FAT	PROTEIN	CARBS
BREAKFAST				
LUNCH				
DINNER				
SNACKS				

HYDRATION

SUPPLEMENTS
☺

HOURS SLEPT LAST NIGHT
Z Z Z Z Z Z Z +

EXERCISE

	TIME	DISTANCE	WEIGHT	REPS	SETS
ACTIVITY 1					
ACTIVITY 2					
ACTIVITY 3					
ACTIVITY 4					

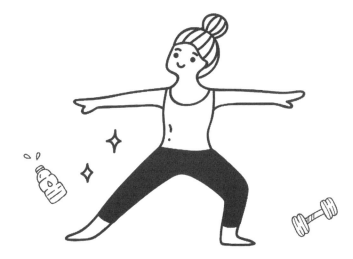

Mind & Spirit

PRAYER/MEDITATION 🙏

Reflections:

_____

_____

_____

_____

SELF - CARE 🖤

I looked after me by:

_____

_____

_____

_____

GRATITUDE ⭐

I am grateful for:

_____

_____

_____

_____

TODAY I FEEL 😲 🙂 😢 😐 😠

_____

_____

Taking Care of Body.

DATE: _____   S M T W T F S

TODAY'S GOALS

MEALS

	CALORIES	FAT	PROTEIN	CARBS
BREAKFAST				
LUNCH				
DINNER				
SNACKS				

HYDRATION

SUPPLEMENTS
☺

HOURS SLEPT LAST NIGHT
Z Z Z Z Z Z Z ✚

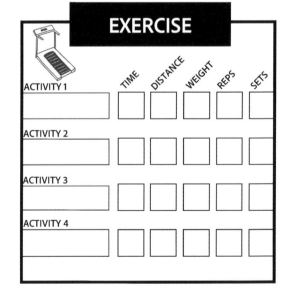

EXERCISE

	TIME	DISTANCE	WEIGHT	REPS	SETS
ACTIVITY 1					
ACTIVITY 2					
ACTIVITY 3					
ACTIVITY 4					

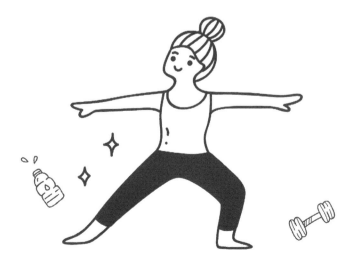

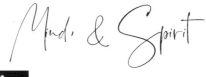

Mind & Spirit

PRAYER/MEDITATION 🙏

Reflections:

_____

_____

_____

SELF - CARE 💙

I looked after me by:

_____

_____

_____

GRATITUDE ⭐

I am grateful for:

_____

_____

_____

TODAY I FEEL 😮 🙂 😢 😐 😠

_____

_____

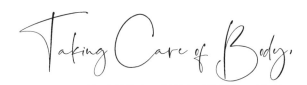

Taking Care of Body,

DATE: _____   S M T W T F S

TODAY'S GOALS

MEALS

	CALORIES	FAT	PROTEIN	CARBS
BREAKFAST				
LUNCH				
DINNER				
SNACKS				

HYDRATION

SUPPLEMENTS

☺

HOURS SLEPT LAST NIGHT

Z Z Z Z Z Z Z +

EXERCISE

	TIME	DISTANCE	WEIGHT	REPS	SETS
ACTIVITY 1					
ACTIVITY 2					
ACTIVITY 3					
ACTIVITY 4					

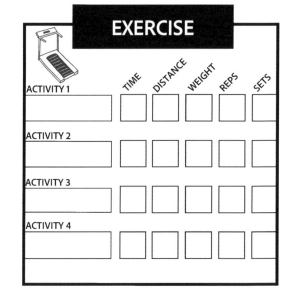

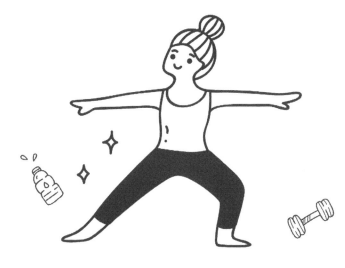

Mind & Spirit

PRAYER/MEDITATION 🙏

Reflections:

_____

_____

_____

_____

SELF - CARE 🖤

I looked after me by:

_____

_____

_____

_____

GRATITUDE ✦

I am grateful for:

_____

_____

_____

_____

TODAY I FEEL 😮 🙂 🥺 😐 😠

_____

_____

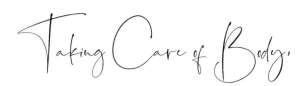

Taking Care of Body

DATE: _____   S M T W T F S

TODAY'S GOALS

MEALS

	CALORIES	FAT	PROTEIN	CARBS
BREAKFAST				
LUNCH				
DINNER				
SNACKS				

HYDRATION

SUPPLEMENTS

☺

HOURS SLEPT LAST NIGHT

Z Z Z Z Z Z Z +

EXERCISE

	TIME	DISTANCE	WEIGHT	REPS	SETS
ACTIVITY 1					
ACTIVITY 2					
ACTIVITY 3					
ACTIVITY 4					

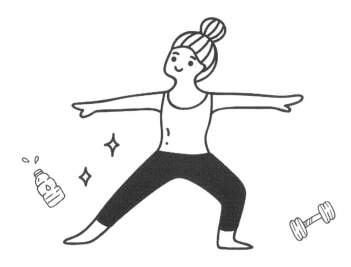

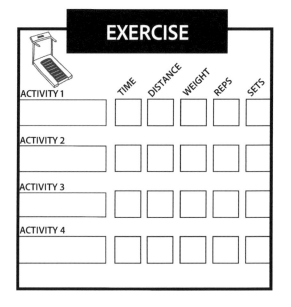

Mind & Spirit

PRAYER/MEDITATION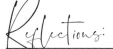

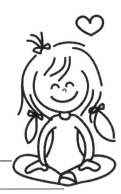

Reflections:

_____

_____

_____

_____

SELF - CARE ♥

I looked after me by:

_____

_____

_____

_____

GRATITUDE ⭐

I am grateful for:

_____

_____

_____

_____

TODAY I FEEL 😲 🙂 😢 😐 😠

_____

_____

Taking Care of Body,

DATE: _____   S M T W T F S

TODAY'S GOALS

MEALS

	CALORIES	FAT	PROTEIN	CARBS
BREAKFAST				
LUNCH				
DINNER				
SNACKS				

HYDRATION

SUPPLEMENTS

☺

HOURS SLEPT LAST NIGHT

Z Z Z Z Z Z Z +

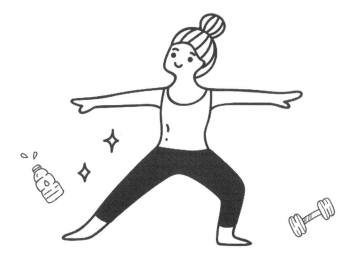

EXERCISE

	TIME	DISTANCE	WEIGHT	REPS	SETS
ACTIVITY 1					
ACTIVITY 2					
ACTIVITY 3					
ACTIVITY 4					

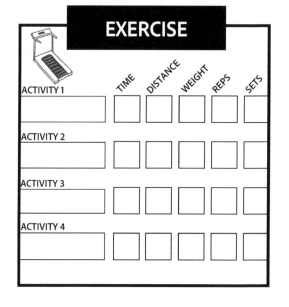

Mind & Spirit

PRAYER/MEDITATION 🙏

Reflections:

_____
_____
_____
_____

SELF - CARE 🖤

I looked after me by:

_____
_____
_____
_____

GRATITUDE ⭐

I am grateful for:

_____
_____
_____
_____

TODAY I FEEL 😲 🙂 😢 😐 😠

_____
_____

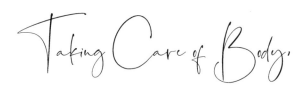

DATE: _____   S M T W T F S

TODAY'S GOALS

MEALS

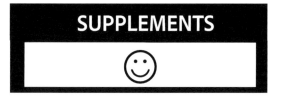

	CALORIES	FAT	PROTEIN	CARBS
BREAKFAST				
LUNCH				
DINNER				
SNACKS				

HYDRATION

SUPPLEMENTS

☺

HOURS SLEPT LAST NIGHT

Z Z Z Z Z Z Z +

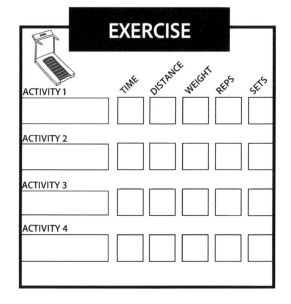

EXERCISE

	TIME	DISTANCE	WEIGHT	REPS	SETS
ACTIVITY 1					
ACTIVITY 2					
ACTIVITY 3					
ACTIVITY 4					

Mind & Spirit

PRAYER/MEDITATION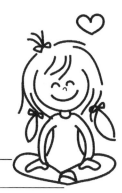

Reflections:

_____

_____

_____

_____

SELF - CARE ♥

I looked after me by:

_____

_____

_____

_____

GRATITUDE ✦

I am grateful for:

_____

_____

_____

_____

TODAY I FEEL 😮 🙂 🥲 😐 😠

_____

_____

Taking Care of Body

DATE: [   ]   S M T W T F S

TODAY'S GOALS

MEALS

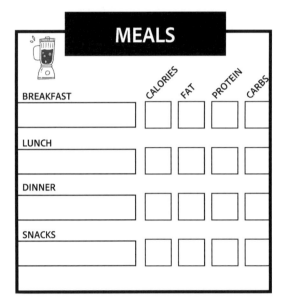

	CALORIES	FAT	PROTEIN	CARBS
BREAKFAST				
LUNCH				
DINNER				
SNACKS				

HYDRATION

SUPPLEMENTS

☺

HOURS SLEPT LAST NIGHT

Z Z Z Z Z Z Z +

EXERCISE

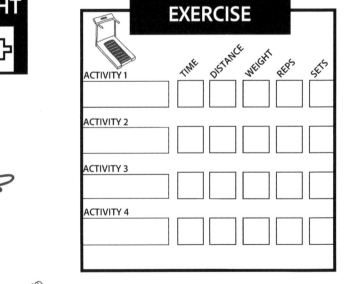

	TIME	DISTANCE	WEIGHT	REPS	SETS
ACTIVITY 1					
ACTIVITY 2					
ACTIVITY 3					
ACTIVITY 4					

Mind & Spirit

PRAYER/MEDITATION 🙏

Reflections:

_____

_____

_____

SELF - CARE ♥

I looked after me by:

_____

_____

_____

GRATITUDE ⭐

I am grateful for:

_____

_____

_____

TODAY I FEEL 😲 🙂 😢 😐 😠

_____

_____

Taking Care of Body

DATE: _____   S M T W T F S

TODAY'S GOALS

MEALS

	CALORIES	FAT	PROTEIN	CARBS
BREAKFAST				
LUNCH				
DINNER				
SNACKS				

HYDRATION

SUPPLEMENTS

:)

HOURS SLEPT LAST NIGHT

Z Z Z Z Z Z Z +

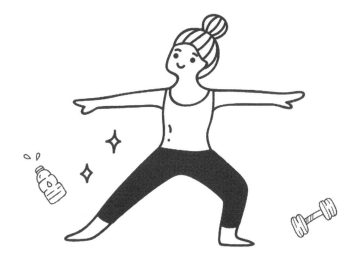

EXERCISE

	TIME	DISTANCE	WEIGHT	REPS	SETS
ACTIVITY 1					
ACTIVITY 2					
ACTIVITY 3					
ACTIVITY 4					

Mind & Spirit

PRAYER/MEDITATION 🙏

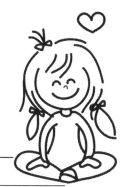

Reflections:

_____

_____

_____

SELF - CARE 🖤

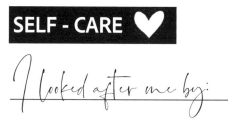

I looked after me by:

_____

_____

_____

GRATITUDE ✮

I am grateful for:

_____

_____

_____

TODAY I FEEL 😲 🙂 😢 😐 😠

_____

_____

Taking Care of Body,

DATE: [   ]   S M T W T F S

TODAY'S GOALS

MEALS

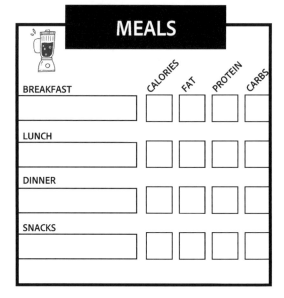

	CALORIES	FAT	PROTEIN	CARBS
BREAKFAST				
LUNCH				
DINNER				
SNACKS				

HYDRATION

SUPPLEMENTS

☺

HOURS SLEPT LAST NIGHT

Z Z Z Z Z Z Z ✛

EXERCISE

	TIME	DISTANCE	WEIGHT	REPS	SETS
ACTIVITY 1					
ACTIVITY 2					
ACTIVITY 3					
ACTIVITY 4					

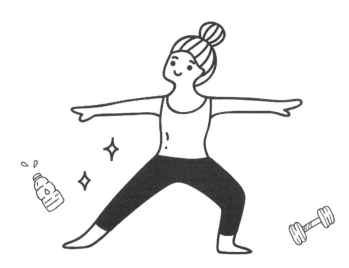

Mind & Spirit

PRAYER/MEDITATION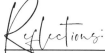

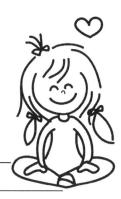

Reflections:

_____

_____

_____

SELF - CARE ♥

I looked after me by:

_____

_____

_____

GRATITUDE ⭐

I am grateful for:

_____

_____

_____

TODAY I FEEL 😲 🙂 😢 😐 😠

_____

_____

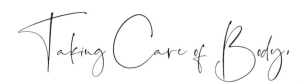

DATE: _____ 　　　　　S M T W T F S

TODAY'S GOALS

MEALS

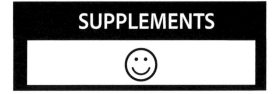

	CALORIES	FAT	PROTEIN	CARBS
BREAKFAST				
LUNCH				
DINNER				
SNACKS				

HYDRATION

SUPPLEMENTS

☺

HOURS SLEPT LAST NIGHT

Z Z Z Z Z Z Z +

EXERCISE

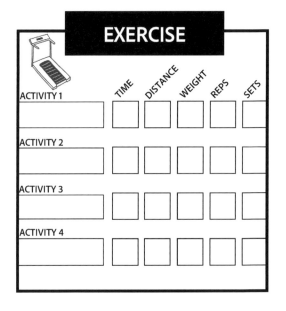

	TIME	DISTANCE	WEIGHT	REPS	SETS
ACTIVITY 1					
ACTIVITY 2					
ACTIVITY 3					
ACTIVITY 4					

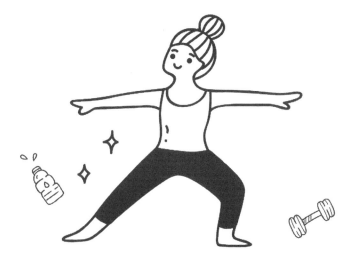

Mind & Spirit

PRAYER/MEDITATION 🙏

Reflections:

_____
_____
_____
_____

SELF - CARE 🖤

I looked after me by:

_____
_____
_____
_____

GRATITUDE ⭐

I am grateful for:

_____
_____
_____
_____

TODAY I FEEL 😮 🙂 🥺 😐 😠

_____
_____

Taking Care of Body,

DATE: [   ] S M T W T F S

TODAY'S GOALS

MEALS

	CALORIES	FAT	PROTEIN	CARBS
BREAKFAST				
LUNCH				
DINNER				
SNACKS				

HYDRATION

SUPPLEMENTS

☺

HOURS SLEPT LAST NIGHT

Z Z Z Z Z Z Z +

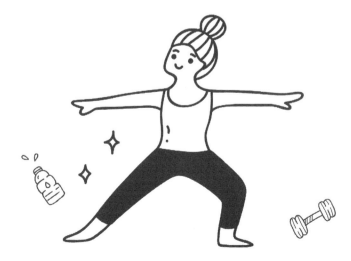

EXERCISE

	TIME	DISTANCE	WEIGHT	REPS	SETS
ACTIVITY 1					
ACTIVITY 2					
ACTIVITY 3					
ACTIVITY 4					

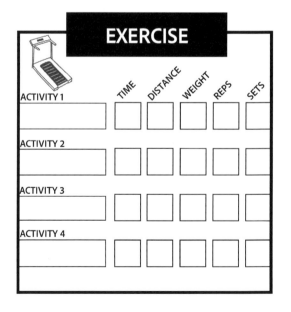

Mind & Spirit

PRAYER/MEDITATION 🙏

Reflections: _____

_____
_____
_____

SELF - CARE 🤍

I looked after me by: _____

_____
_____
_____

GRATITUDE ⭐

I am grateful for: _____

_____
_____
_____

TODAY I FEEL 😮 🙂 🥺 😐 😠

_____
_____

Taking Care of Body,

DATE: _____   S M T W T F S

TODAY'S GOALS

MEALS

	CALORIES	FAT	PROTEIN	CARBS
BREAKFAST				
LUNCH				
DINNER				
SNACKS				

HYDRATION

🥤 🥤 🥤 🥤 🥤 🥤 🥤 🥤

SUPPLEMENTS

☺

HOURS SLEPT LAST NIGHT

Z Z Z Z Z Z Z +

EXERCISE

	TIME	DISTANCE	WEIGHT	REPS	SETS
ACTIVITY 1					
ACTIVITY 2					
ACTIVITY 3					
ACTIVITY 4					

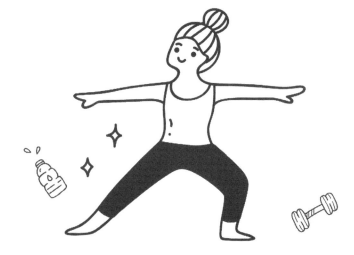

Mind & Spirit

PRAYER/MEDITATION 🙏

Reflections:

_____
_____
_____

SELF - CARE ♥

I looked after me by:

_____
_____
_____

GRATITUDE ⭐

I am grateful for:

_____
_____
_____

TODAY I FEEL 😮 🙂 🥺 😐 😠

_____
_____

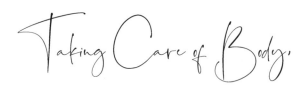

Taking Care of Body

DATE: [   ]   S M T W T F S

TODAY'S GOALS

MEALS

	CALORIES	FAT	PROTEIN	CARBS
BREAKFAST				
LUNCH				
DINNER				
SNACKS				

HYDRATION

SUPPLEMENTS

☺

HOURS SLEPT LAST NIGHT

ZZZZZZZ+

EXERCISE

	TIME	DISTANCE	WEIGHT	REPS	SETS
ACTIVITY 1					
ACTIVITY 2					
ACTIVITY 3					
ACTIVITY 4					

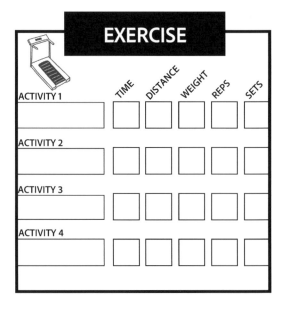

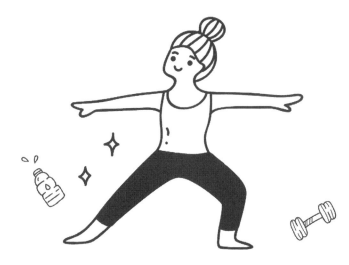

Mind & Spirit

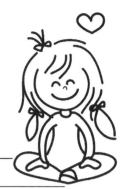

PRAYER/MEDITATION 🙏

Reflections:

_____

_____

_____

SELF - CARE 🖤

I looked after me by:

_____

_____

_____

GRATITUDE ✫

I am grateful for:

_____

_____

_____

TODAY I FEEL 😲 🙂 😢 😐 😠

_____

_____

Taking Care of Body,

DATE: _____   S M T W T F S

TODAY'S GOALS

MEALS

	CALORIES	FAT	PROTEIN	CARBS
BREAKFAST				
LUNCH				
DINNER				
SNACKS				

HYDRATION

SUPPLEMENTS

☺

HOURS SLEPT LAST NIGHT

Z Z Z Z Z Z Z +

EXERCISE

	TIME	DISTANCE	WEIGHT	REPS	SETS
ACTIVITY 1					
ACTIVITY 2					
ACTIVITY 3					
ACTIVITY 4					

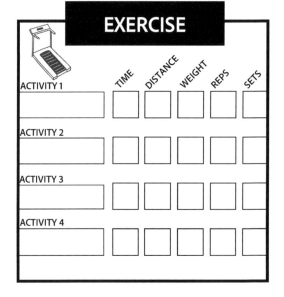

Mind & Spirit

PRAYER/MEDITATION 🙏

Reflections:

_____

_____
_____
_____

SELF - CARE 🖤

I looked after me by:

_____
_____
_____
_____

GRATITUDE ⭐

I am grateful for:

_____
_____
_____
_____

TODAY I FEEL 😲 🙂 🥹 😐 😠

_____
_____

Taking Care of Body.

DATE: _____   S M T W T F S

TODAY'S GOALS

MEALS

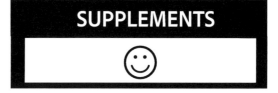

	CALORIES	FAT	PROTEIN	CARBS
BREAKFAST				
LUNCH				
DINNER				
SNACKS				

HYDRATION

SUPPLEMENTS

☺

HOURS SLEPT LAST NIGHT

Z Z Z Z Z Z Z +

EXERCISE

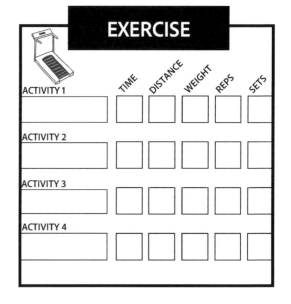

	TIME	DISTANCE	WEIGHT	REPS	SETS
ACTIVITY 1					
ACTIVITY 2					
ACTIVITY 3					
ACTIVITY 4					

Mind & Spirit

PRAYER/MEDITATION 🙏

Reflections:

_____

_____

_____

_____

SELF - CARE 🖤

I looked after me by:

_____

_____

_____

_____

GRATITUDE ⭐

I am grateful for:

_____

_____

_____

_____

TODAY I FEEL 😮 🙂 😢 😐 😠

_____

_____

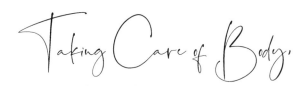

Taking Care of Body,

DATE: _____   **S M T W T F S**

TODAY'S GOALS

MEALS

	CALORIES	FAT	PROTEIN	CARBS
BREAKFAST				
LUNCH				
DINNER				
SNACKS				

HYDRATION

SUPPLEMENTS

:)

HOURS SLEPT LAST NIGHT

Z Z Z Z Z Z Z +

EXERCISE

	TIME	DISTANCE	WEIGHT	REPS	SETS
ACTIVITY 1					
ACTIVITY 2					
ACTIVITY 3					
ACTIVITY 4					

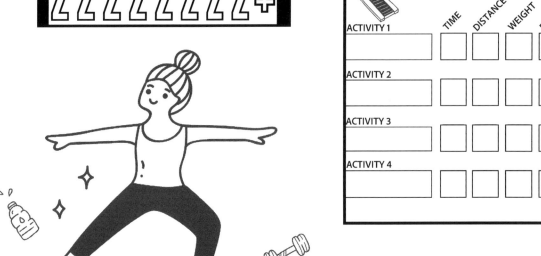

Mind & Spirit

PRAYER/MEDITATION 🙏

Reflections:

_____

_____

_____

SELF - CARE 💙

I looked after me by:

_____

_____

_____

_____

GRATITUDE ⭐

I am grateful for:

_____

_____

_____

_____

TODAY I FEEL 😲 🙂 😢 😐 😠

_____

_____

Taking Care of Body,

DATE: [   ]   S M T W T F S

TODAY'S GOALS

MEALS

	CALORIES	FAT	PROTEIN	CARBS
BREAKFAST				
LUNCH				
DINNER				
SNACKS				

HYDRATION

SUPPLEMENTS

☺

HOURS SLEPT LAST NIGHT

ZZZZZZZ+

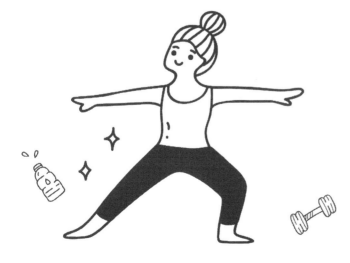

EXERCISE

	TIME	DISTANCE	WEIGHT	REPS	SETS
ACTIVITY 1					
ACTIVITY 2					
ACTIVITY 3					
ACTIVITY 4					

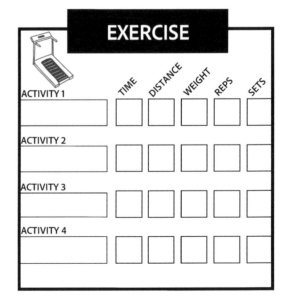

Mind & Spirit

PRAYER/MEDITATION 🙏

Reflections:

_____
_____
_____
_____

SELF - CARE 🖤

I looked after me by:

_____
_____
_____
_____

GRATITUDE ⭐

I am grateful for:

_____
_____
_____
_____

TODAY I FEEL 😲 🙂 🥺 😐 😠

_____
_____

Taking Care of Body.

DATE: _____   S M T W T F S

TODAY'S GOALS

MEALS

	CALORIES	FAT	PROTEIN	CARBS
BREAKFAST				
LUNCH				
DINNER				
SNACKS				

HYDRATION

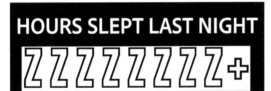

SUPPLEMENTS

☺

HOURS SLEPT LAST NIGHT

Z Z Z Z Z Z Z +

EXERCISE

	TIME	DISTANCE	WEIGHT	REPS	SETS
ACTIVITY 1					
ACTIVITY 2					
ACTIVITY 3					
ACTIVITY 4					

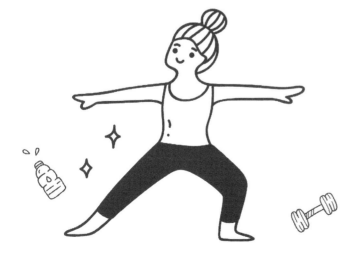

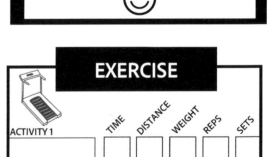

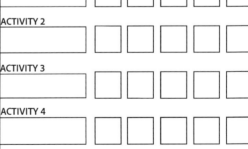

Mind & Spirit

PRAYER/MEDITATION 🙏

Reflections:

_____

_____

_____

SELF - CARE 🖤

I looked after me by:

_____

_____

_____

GRATITUDE ⭐

I am grateful for:

_____

_____

_____

TODAY I FEEL 😲 🙂 😢 😐 😠

_____

_____

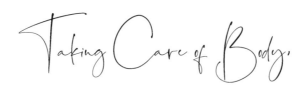

Taking Care of Body.

DATE:

TODAY'S GOALS

MEALS

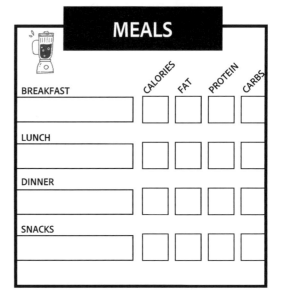

	CALORIES	FAT	PROTEIN	CARBS
BREAKFAST				
LUNCH				
DINNER				
SNACKS				

HYDRATION

SUPPLEMENTS

HOURS SLEPT LAST NIGHT

Z Z Z Z Z Z Z +

EXERCISE

	TIME	DISTANCE	WEIGHT	REPS	SETS
ACTIVITY 1					
ACTIVITY 2					
ACTIVITY 3					
ACTIVITY 4					

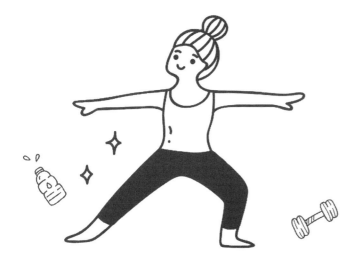

Mind & Spirit

PRAYER/MEDITATION 🙏

Reflections:

_____

_____

_____

_____

SELF - CARE 💜

I looked after me by:

_____

_____

_____

_____

GRATITUDE ⭐

I am grateful for:

_____

_____

_____

_____

TODAY I FEEL 😲 🙂 😢 😐 😠

_____

_____

Taking Care of Body

DATE: _____ S M T W T F S

TODAY'S GOALS

MEALS

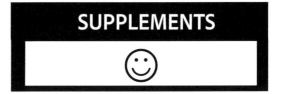

	CALORIES	FAT	PROTEIN	CARBS
BREAKFAST				
LUNCH				
DINNER				
SNACKS				

HYDRATION

SUPPLEMENTS

:)

HOURS SLEPT LAST NIGHT

Z Z Z Z Z Z Z +

EXERCISE

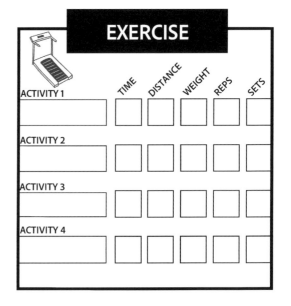

	TIME	DISTANCE	WEIGHT	REPS	SETS
ACTIVITY 1					
ACTIVITY 2					
ACTIVITY 3					
ACTIVITY 4					

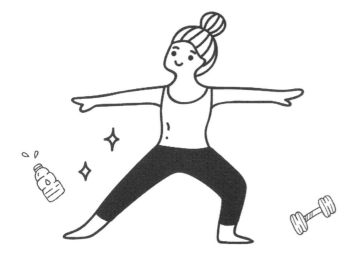

Mind & Spirit

PRAYER/MEDITATION 🙏

Reflections:

_____

_____
_____
_____

SELF - CARE 🖤

I looked after me by:

_____
_____
_____
_____

GRATITUDE ⭐

I am grateful for:

_____
_____
_____
_____

TODAY I FEEL 😮 🙂 😢 😐 😠

_____

_____

Taking Care of Body,

DATE: [_____]   S M T W T F S

TODAY'S GOALS

MEALS

	CALORIES	FAT	PROTEIN	CARBS
BREAKFAST				
LUNCH				
DINNER				
SNACKS				

HYDRATION

SUPPLEMENTS

☺

HOURS SLEPT LAST NIGHT

Z Z Z Z Z Z Z +

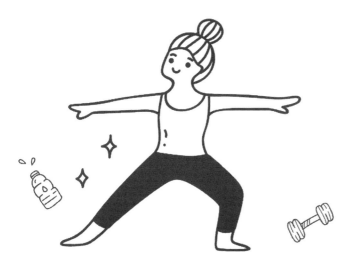

EXERCISE

	TIME	DISTANCE	WEIGHT	REPS	SETS
ACTIVITY 1					
ACTIVITY 2					
ACTIVITY 3					
ACTIVITY 4					

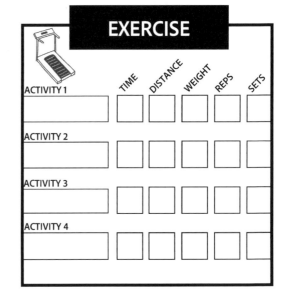

Mind & Spirit

PRAYER/MEDITATION 🙏

Reflections:

_____

_____
_____
_____

SELF - CARE 🖤

I looked after me by:

_____
_____
_____
_____

GRATITUDE ⭐

I am grateful for:

_____
_____
_____
_____

TODAY I FEEL 😲 🙂 😢 😐 😠

_____
_____

Taking Care of Body,

DATE: _____   S M T W T F S

TODAY'S GOALS

MEALS

	CALORIES	FAT	PROTEIN	CARBS
BREAKFAST				
LUNCH				
DINNER				
SNACKS				

HYDRATION

SUPPLEMENTS

HOURS SLEPT LAST NIGHT

ZZZZZZZ+

EXERCISE

	TIME	DISTANCE	WEIGHT	REPS	SETS
ACTIVITY 1					
ACTIVITY 2					
ACTIVITY 3					
ACTIVITY 4					

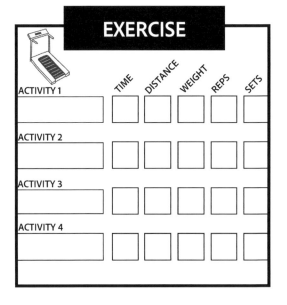

Mind, & Spirit

PRAYER/MEDITATION 🙏

Reflections:

_____

_____

_____

_____

SELF - CARE 🖤

I looked after me by:

_____

_____

_____

_____

GRATITUDE ✦

I am grateful for:

_____

_____

_____

_____

TODAY I FEEL 😲 🙂 🥺 😐 😠

_____

_____

Taking Care of Body,

DATE: _____ S M T W T F S

TODAY'S GOALS

MEALS

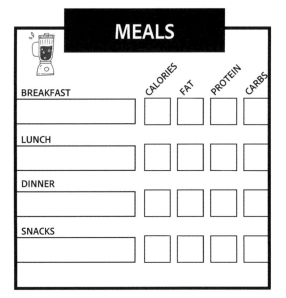

	CALORIES	FAT	PROTEIN	CARBS
BREAKFAST				
LUNCH				
DINNER				
SNACKS				

HYDRATION

SUPPLEMENTS

☺

HOURS SLEPT LAST NIGHT

Z Z Z Z Z Z Z +

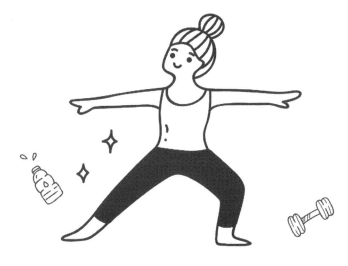

EXERCISE

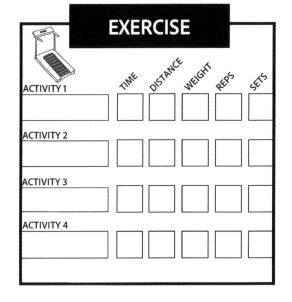

	TIME	DISTANCE	WEIGHT	REPS	SETS
ACTIVITY 1					
ACTIVITY 2					
ACTIVITY 3					
ACTIVITY 4					

Mind & Spirit

PRAYER/MEDITATION 🙏

Reflections:

_____

_____

_____

_____

SELF - CARE 🖤

I looked after me by:

_____

_____

_____

_____

GRATITUDE ✦

I am grateful for:

_____

_____

_____

_____

TODAY I FEEL 😲 🙂 😢 😐 😠

_____

_____

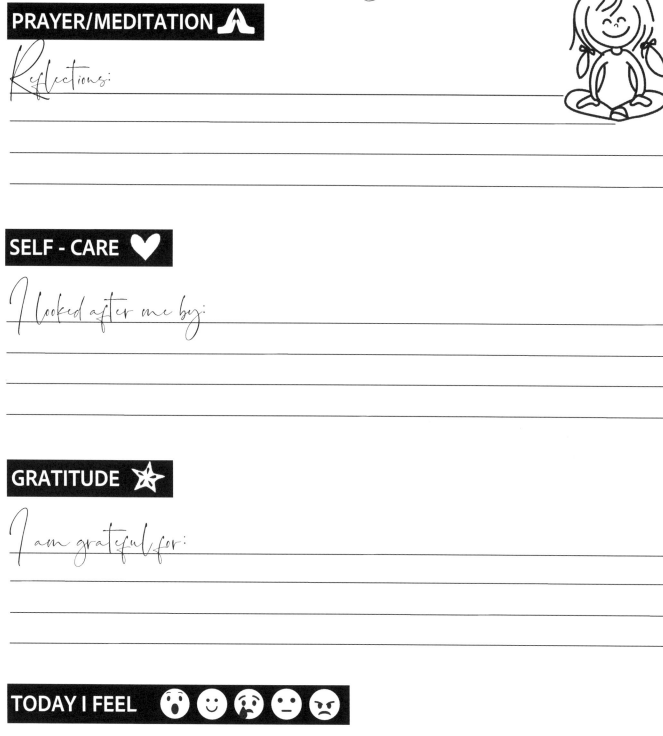

Taking Care of Body,

DATE: _____   S M T W T F S

TODAY'S GOALS

MEALS

	CALORIES	FAT	PROTEIN	CARBS
BREAKFAST				
LUNCH				
DINNER				
SNACKS				

HYDRATION

SUPPLEMENTS

HOURS SLEPT LAST NIGHT

Z Z Z Z Z Z Z +

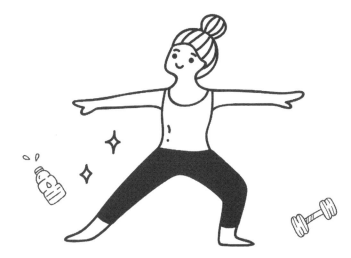

EXERCISE

	TIME	DISTANCE	WEIGHT	REPS	SETS
ACTIVITY 1					
ACTIVITY 2					
ACTIVITY 3					
ACTIVITY 4					

Mind & Spirit

PRAYER/MEDITATION 🙏

Reflections:

_____

_____

_____

_____

SELF - CARE 🖤

I looked after me by:

_____

_____

_____

_____

GRATITUDE ⭐

I am grateful for:

_____

_____

_____

_____

TODAY I FEEL 😮 🙂 😢 😐 😠

_____

_____

Taking Care of Body,

DATE: [_____]   S M T W T F S

TODAY'S GOALS

MEALS

	CALORIES	FAT	PROTEIN	CARBS
BREAKFAST				
LUNCH				
DINNER				
SNACKS				

HYDRATION

SUPPLEMENTS

☺

HOURS SLEPT LAST NIGHT

Z Z Z Z Z Z Z +

EXERCISE

	TIME	DISTANCE	WEIGHT	REPS	SETS
ACTIVITY 1					
ACTIVITY 2					
ACTIVITY 3					
ACTIVITY 4					

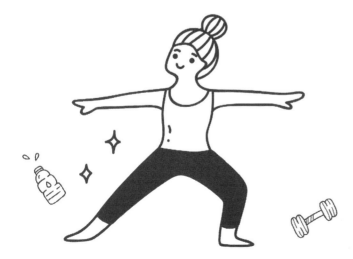

Mind & Spirit

PRAYER/MEDITATION 🙏

Reflections:

_____
_____
_____

SELF - CARE 🖤

I looked after me by:

_____
_____
_____

GRATITUDE ⭐

I am grateful for:

_____
_____
_____

TODAY I FEEL 😮 🙂 😢 😐 😠

_____
_____

Taking Care of Body.

DATE: _____ S M T W T F S

TODAY'S GOALS

MEALS

	CALORIES	FAT	PROTEIN	CARBS
BREAKFAST				
LUNCH				
DINNER				
SNACKS				

HYDRATION

SUPPLEMENTS

🙂

HOURS SLEPT LAST NIGHT

Z Z Z Z Z Z Z ✚

EXERCISE

	TIME	DISTANCE	WEIGHT	REPS	SETS
ACTIVITY 1					
ACTIVITY 2					
ACTIVITY 3					
ACTIVITY 4					

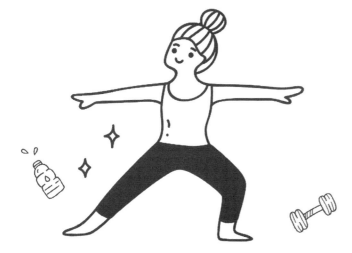

Mind & Spirit

PRAYER/MEDITATION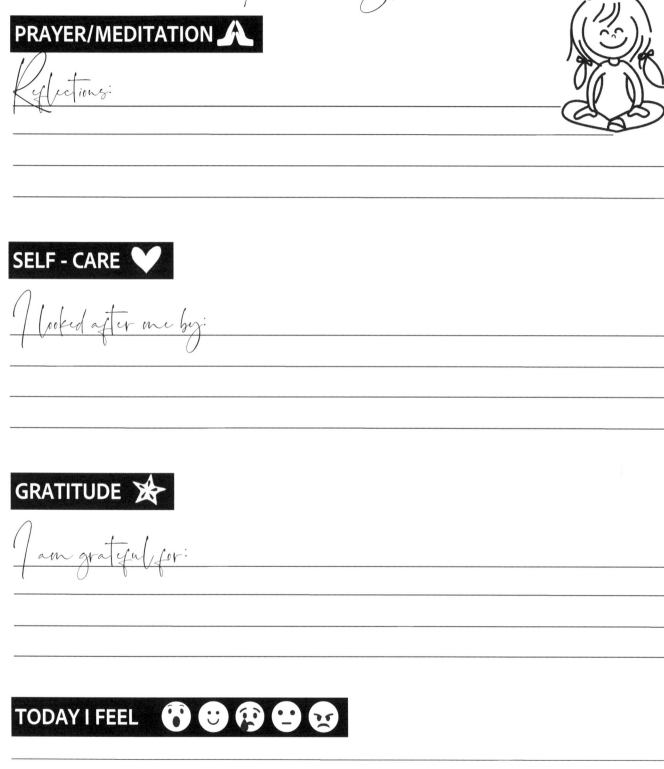

Reflections:

_____

_____

_____

_____

SELF - CARE ♥

I looked after me by:

_____

_____

_____

_____

GRATITUDE ✦

I am grateful for:

_____

_____

_____

_____

TODAY I FEEL 😲 🙂 😢 😐 😠

_____

_____

Taking Care of Body

DATE: _____   S M T W T F S

TODAY'S GOALS

MEALS

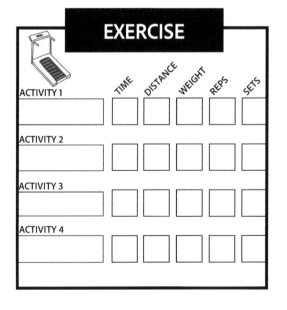

	CALORIES	FAT	PROTEIN	CARBS
BREAKFAST				
LUNCH				
DINNER				
SNACKS				

HYDRATION

SUPPLEMENTS

☺

HOURS SLEPT LAST NIGHT

Z Z Z Z Z Z Z ✚

EXERCISE

	TIME	DISTANCE	WEIGHT	REPS	SETS
ACTIVITY 1					
ACTIVITY 2					
ACTIVITY 3					
ACTIVITY 4					

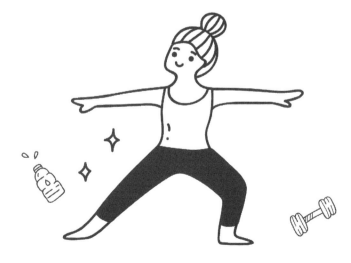

Mind & Spirit

PRAYER/MEDITATION 🙏

Reflections:

_____

_____
_____
_____

SELF - CARE 🖤

I looked after me by:

_____
_____
_____
_____

GRATITUDE ⭐

I am grateful for:

_____
_____
_____
_____

TODAY I FEEL 😮 🙂 😢 😐 😠

_____

_____

Taking Care of Body,

DATE: [   ]   S M T W T F S

TODAY'S GOALS

MEALS

	CALORIES	FAT	PROTEIN	CARBS
BREAKFAST				
LUNCH				
DINNER				
SNACKS				

HYDRATION

SUPPLEMENTS

:)

HOURS SLEPT LAST NIGHT

Z Z Z Z Z Z Z +

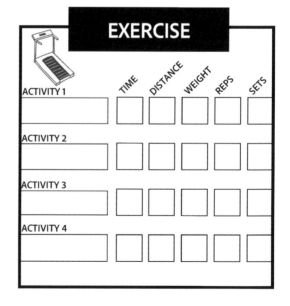

EXERCISE

	TIME	DISTANCE	WEIGHT	REPS	SETS
ACTIVITY 1					
ACTIVITY 2					
ACTIVITY 3					
ACTIVITY 4					

Mind & Spirit

PRAYER/MEDITATION 🙏

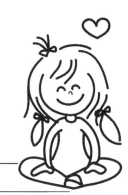

Reflections:

_____

_____

_____

_____

SELF - CARE 🖤

I looked after me by:

_____

_____

_____

_____

GRATITUDE ⭐

I am grateful for:

_____

_____

_____

_____

TODAY I FEEL 😮 🙂 😢 😐 😠

_____

_____

Taking Care of Body

DATE: [_____]   S M T W T F S

TODAY'S GOALS

MEALS

	CALORIES	FAT	PROTEIN	CARBS
BREAKFAST				
LUNCH				
DINNER				
SNACKS				

HYDRATION

SUPPLEMENTS

☺

HOURS SLEPT LAST NIGHT

Z Z Z Z Z Z Z +

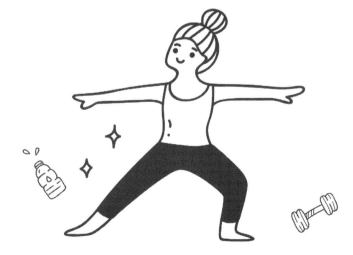

EXERCISE

	TIME	DISTANCE	WEIGHT	REPS	SETS
ACTIVITY 1					
ACTIVITY 2					
ACTIVITY 3					
ACTIVITY 4					

Mind & Spirit

PRAYER/MEDITATION 🙏

Reflections:

_____
_____
_____
_____

SELF - CARE ♥

I looked after me by:

_____
_____
_____
_____

GRATITUDE ⭐

I am grateful for:

_____
_____
_____
_____

TODAY I FEEL 😲 🙂 😢 😐 😠

_____
_____

Taking Care of Body

DATE: [_____]

TODAY'S GOALS

MEALS

	CALORIES	FAT	PROTEIN	CARBS
BREAKFAST				
LUNCH				
DINNER				
SNACKS				

HYDRATION

SUPPLEMENTS

:)

HOURS SLEPT LAST NIGHT

Z Z Z Z Z Z Z +

EXERCISE

	TIME	DISTANCE	WEIGHT	REPS	SETS
ACTIVITY 1					
ACTIVITY 2					
ACTIVITY 3					
ACTIVITY 4					

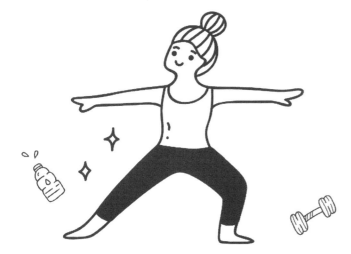

Mind & Spirit

PRAYER/MEDITATION 🙏

Reflections:

_____

_____

_____

SELF - CARE 🖤

I looked after me by:

_____

_____

_____

GRATITUDE ⭐

I am grateful for:

_____

_____

_____

TODAY I FEEL 😲 🙂 😢 😐 😠

_____

_____

Taking Care of Body,

DATE: _____   S M T W T F S

TODAY'S GOALS

MEALS

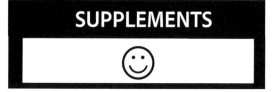

	CALORIES	FAT	PROTEIN	CARBS
BREAKFAST				
LUNCH				
DINNER				
SNACKS				

HYDRATION

SUPPLEMENTS

😊

HOURS SLEPT LAST NIGHT

Z Z Z Z Z Z Z +

EXERCISE

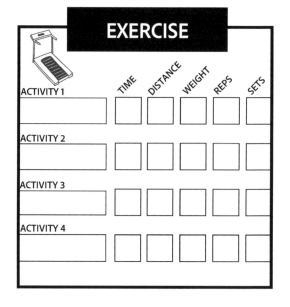

	TIME	DISTANCE	WEIGHT	REPS	SETS
ACTIVITY 1					
ACTIVITY 2					
ACTIVITY 3					
ACTIVITY 4					

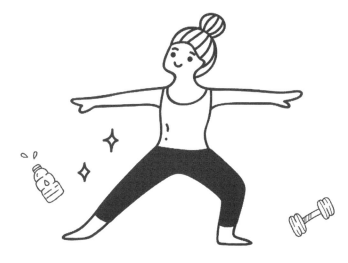

Mind, & Spirit

PRAYER/MEDITATION 🙏

Reflections:

_____

_____
_____
_____

SELF - CARE 🖤

I looked after me by:

_____

_____
_____
_____

GRATITUDE ⭐

I am grateful for:

_____

_____
_____
_____

TODAY I FEEL 😮 🙂 😢 😐 😠

_____

_____

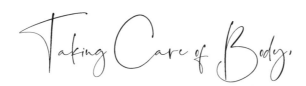

Taking Care of Body.

DATE: _____   S M T W T F S

TODAY'S GOALS

_____
_____
_____
_____
_____
_____
_____
_____

MEALS

	CALORIES	FAT	PROTEIN	CARBS
BREAKFAST				
LUNCH				
DINNER				
SNACKS				

HYDRATION

SUPPLEMENTS
:)

HOURS SLEPT LAST NIGHT
ZZZZZZZ+

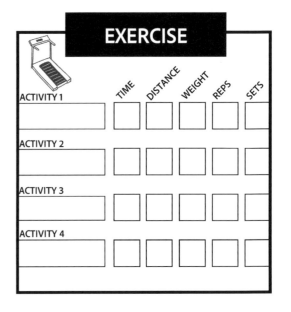

EXERCISE

	TIME	DISTANCE	WEIGHT	REPS	SETS
ACTIVITY 1					
ACTIVITY 2					
ACTIVITY 3					
ACTIVITY 4					

Mind & Spirit

PRAYER/MEDITATION 🙏

Reflections:

_____

_____

_____

SELF - CARE ❤️

I looked after me by:

_____

_____

_____

GRATITUDE ⭐

I am grateful for:

_____

_____

_____

TODAY I FEEL 😮 🙂 🥺 😐 😠

_____

_____

Taking Care of Body,

DATE: [   ]   S M T W T F S

TODAY'S GOALS

MEALS

	CALORIES	FAT	PROTEIN	CARBS
BREAKFAST				
LUNCH				
DINNER				
SNACKS				

HYDRATION

SUPPLEMENTS

☺

HOURS SLEPT LAST NIGHT

Z Z Z Z Z Z Z +

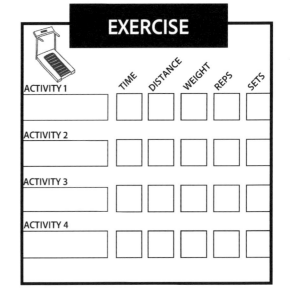

EXERCISE

	TIME	DISTANCE	WEIGHT	REPS	SETS
ACTIVITY 1					
ACTIVITY 2					
ACTIVITY 3					
ACTIVITY 4					

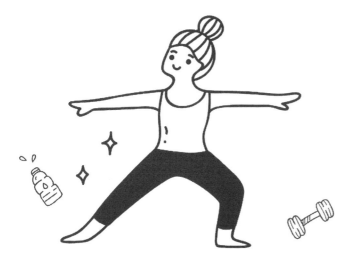

Mind & Spirit

PRAYER/MEDITATION 🙏

Reflections:

_____

_____

_____

_____

SELF - CARE ♥

I looked after me by:

_____

_____

_____

_____

GRATITUDE ✯

I am grateful for:

_____

_____

_____

_____

TODAY I FEEL 😮 🙂 😢 😐 😠

_____

_____

Taking Care of Body

DATE: _____   S M T W T F S

TODAY'S GOALS

MEALS

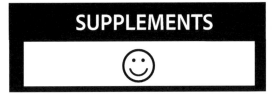

	CALORIES	FAT	PROTEIN	CARBS
BREAKFAST				
LUNCH				
DINNER				
SNACKS				

HYDRATION

SUPPLEMENTS

☺

HOURS SLEPT LAST NIGHT

Z Z Z Z Z Z Z +

EXERCISE

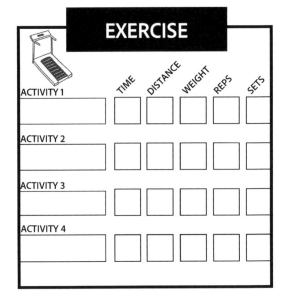

	TIME	DISTANCE	WEIGHT	REPS	SETS
ACTIVITY 1					
ACTIVITY 2					
ACTIVITY 3					
ACTIVITY 4					

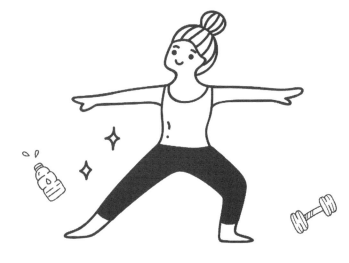

Mind & Spirit

PRAYER/MEDITATION 🙏

Reflections:

_____
_____
_____

SELF - CARE 🖤

I looked after me by:

_____
_____
_____

GRATITUDE ⭐

I am grateful for:

_____
_____
_____

TODAY I FEEL 😮 🙂 😢 😐 😠

_____
_____

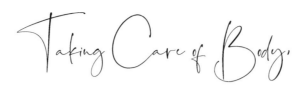

DATE:

TODAY'S GOALS

MEALS

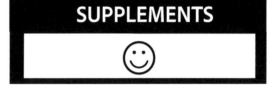

	CALORIES	FAT	PROTEIN	CARBS
BREAKFAST				
LUNCH				
DINNER				
SNACKS				

HYDRATION

SUPPLEMENTS

:)

HOURS SLEPT LAST NIGHT

Z Z Z Z Z Z Z +

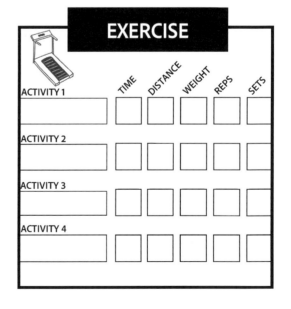

EXERCISE

	TIME	DISTANCE	WEIGHT	REPS	SETS
ACTIVITY 1					
ACTIVITY 2					
ACTIVITY 3					
ACTIVITY 4					

Mind & Spirit

PRAYER/MEDITATION 🙏

Reflections:

_____

_____

_____

SELF - CARE 🤍

I looked after me by:

_____

_____

_____

GRATITUDE ⭐

I am grateful for:

_____

_____

_____

TODAY I FEEL 😮 🙂 😢 😐 😠

_____

_____

Taking Care of Body.

DATE: [_____] S M T W T F S

TODAY'S GOALS

MEALS

	CALORIES	FAT	PROTEIN	CARBS
BREAKFAST				
LUNCH				
DINNER				
SNACKS				

HYDRATION

SUPPLEMENTS
:)

HOURS SLEPT LAST NIGHT
Z Z Z Z Z Z Z +

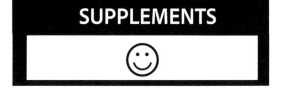

EXERCISE

	TIME	DISTANCE	WEIGHT	REPS	SETS
ACTIVITY 1					
ACTIVITY 2					
ACTIVITY 3					
ACTIVITY 4					

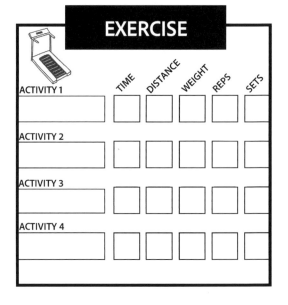

Mind & Spirit

PRAYER/MEDITATION 🙏

Reflections:

_____

_____

_____

_____

SELF - CARE 💜

I looked after me by:

_____

_____

_____

_____

GRATITUDE ⭐

I am grateful for:

_____

_____

_____

_____

TODAY I FEEL 😮 🙂 🥺 😐 😠

_____

_____

Taking Care of Body,

DATE: [   ]   S M T W T F S

TODAY'S GOALS

MEALS

	CALORIES	FAT	PROTEIN	CARBS
BREAKFAST				
LUNCH				
DINNER				
SNACKS				

HYDRATION

SUPPLEMENTS
☺

HOURS SLEPT LAST NIGHT
Z Z Z Z Z Z Z Z +

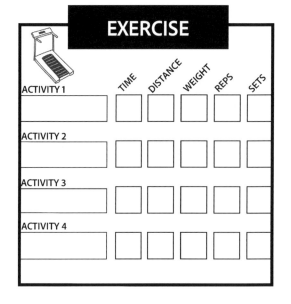

EXERCISE

	TIME	DISTANCE	WEIGHT	REPS	SETS
ACTIVITY 1					
ACTIVITY 2					
ACTIVITY 3					
ACTIVITY 4					

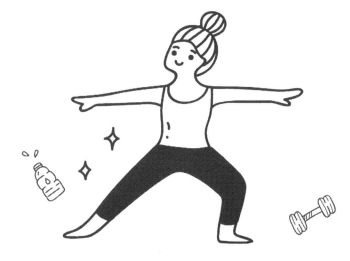

Mind & Spirit

PRAYER/MEDITATION 🙏

Reflections:

_____

_____
_____
_____

SELF - CARE 💜

I looked after me by:

_____

_____
_____
_____

GRATITUDE ⭐

I am grateful for:

_____

_____
_____
_____

TODAY I FEEL 😮 🙂 🥺 😐 😠

_____

_____

Taking Care of Body.

DATE: [   ]   S M T W T F S

TODAY'S GOALS

MEALS

	CALORIES	FAT	PROTEIN	CARBS
BREAKFAST				
LUNCH				
DINNER				
SNACKS				

HYDRATION

SUPPLEMENTS

:)

HOURS SLEPT LAST NIGHT

Z Z Z Z Z Z Z +

EXERCISE

	TIME	DISTANCE	WEIGHT	REPS	SETS
ACTIVITY 1					
ACTIVITY 2					
ACTIVITY 3					
ACTIVITY 4					

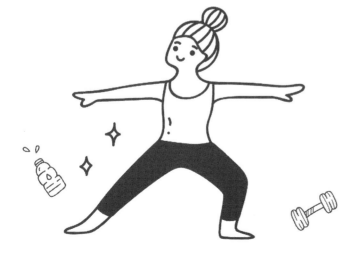

Mind & Spirit

PRAYER/MEDITATION 🙏

Reflections:

_____

_____

_____

_____

SELF - CARE 🖤

I looked after me by:

_____

_____

_____

_____

GRATITUDE ⭐

I am grateful for:

_____

_____

_____

_____

TODAY I FEEL 😮 🙂 😢 😐 😠

_____

_____

Taking Care of Body,

DATE: [_____] S M T W T F S

TODAY'S GOALS

MEALS

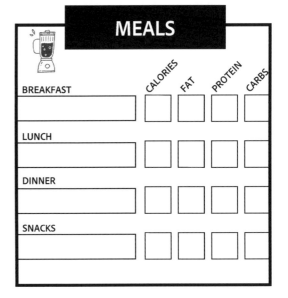

	CALORIES	FAT	PROTEIN	CARBS
BREAKFAST				
LUNCH				
DINNER				
SNACKS				

HYDRATION

SUPPLEMENTS

☺

HOURS SLEPT LAST NIGHT

Z Z Z Z Z Z Z +

EXERCISE

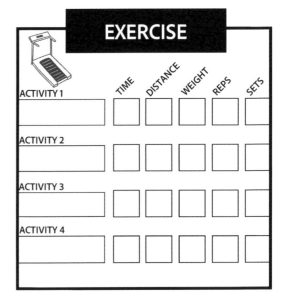

	TIME	DISTANCE	WEIGHT	REPS	SETS
ACTIVITY 1					
ACTIVITY 2					
ACTIVITY 3					
ACTIVITY 4					

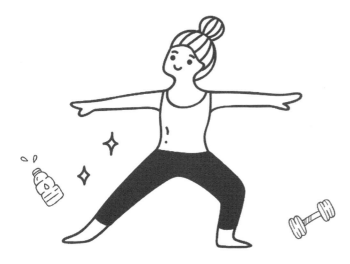

Mind & Spirit

PRAYER/MEDITATION 🙏

Reflections:

_____

_____
_____
_____

SELF - CARE 🖤

I looked after me by:

_____

_____
_____
_____

GRATITUDE ⭐

I am grateful for:

_____

_____
_____
_____

TODAY I FEEL 😲 🙂 😢 😐 😠

_____

_____

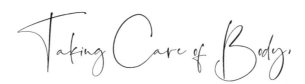

Taking Care of Body

DATE: _____   S M T W T F S

TODAY'S GOALS

MEALS

	CALORIES	FAT	PROTEIN	CARBS
BREAKFAST				
LUNCH				
DINNER				
SNACKS				

HYDRATION

SUPPLEMENTS

🙂

HOURS SLEPT LAST NIGHT

Z Z Z Z Z Z Z ✚

EXERCISE

	TIME	DISTANCE	WEIGHT	REPS	SETS
ACTIVITY 1					
ACTIVITY 2					
ACTIVITY 3					
ACTIVITY 4					

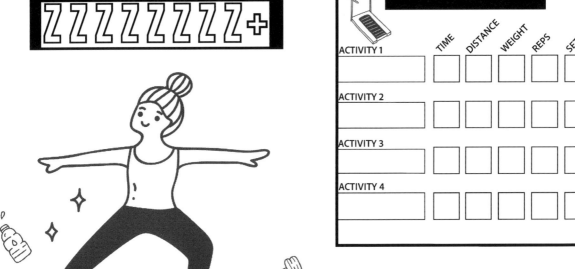

Mind & Spirit

PRAYER/MEDITATION 🙏

Reflections:

_____

_____

_____

_____

SELF - CARE 🖤

I looked after me by:

_____

_____

_____

GRATITUDE ⭐

I am grateful for:

_____

_____

_____

TODAY I FEEL 😮 🙂 😢 😐 😠

_____

_____

Taking Care of Body.

DATE: [   ]   S   M   T   W   T   F   S

TODAY'S GOALS

MEALS

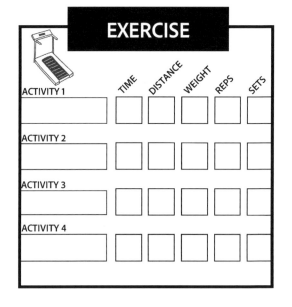

	CALORIES	FAT	PROTEIN	CARBS
BREAKFAST				
LUNCH				
DINNER				
SNACKS				

HYDRATION

SUPPLEMENTS

:)

HOURS SLEPT LAST NIGHT

Z Z Z Z Z Z Z +

EXERCISE

	TIME	DISTANCE	WEIGHT	REPS	SETS
ACTIVITY 1					
ACTIVITY 2					
ACTIVITY 3					
ACTIVITY 4					

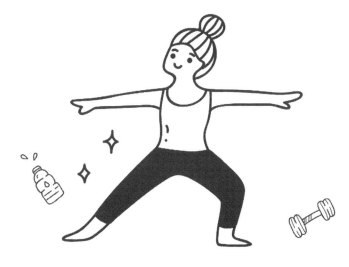

Mind & Spirit

PRAYER/MEDITATION 🙏

Reflections:

_____

_____

_____

_____

SELF - CARE 🖤

I looked after me by:

_____

_____

_____

_____

GRATITUDE ⭐

I am grateful for:

_____

_____

_____

_____

TODAY I FEEL 😲 🙂 😢 😐 😠

_____

_____

Taking Care of Body.

DATE: _____   S M T W T F S

TODAY'S GOALS

MEALS

	CALORIES	FAT	PROTEIN	CARBS
BREAKFAST				
LUNCH				
DINNER				
SNACKS				

HYDRATION

SUPPLEMENTS
:)

HOURS SLEPT LAST NIGHT
ZZZZZZZ+

EXERCISE

	TIME	DISTANCE	WEIGHT	REPS	SETS
ACTIVITY 1					
ACTIVITY 2					
ACTIVITY 3					
ACTIVITY 4					

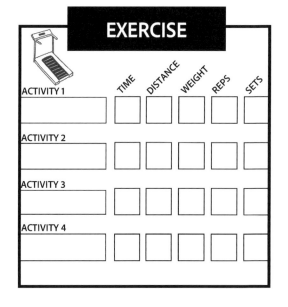

Mind & Spirit

PRAYER/MEDITATION

Reflections:

_____
_____
_____
_____

SELF - CARE ♥

I looked after me by:

_____
_____
_____
_____

GRATITUDE ✦

I am grateful for:

_____
_____
_____
_____

TODAY I FEEL 😮 🙂 😢 😐 😠

_____
_____

Taking Care of Body.

DATE: ⬚⬚⬚⬚⬚⬚⬚⬚⬚⬚⬚⬚⬚⬚⬚⬚⬚   S M T W T F S

TODAY'S GOALS

MEALS

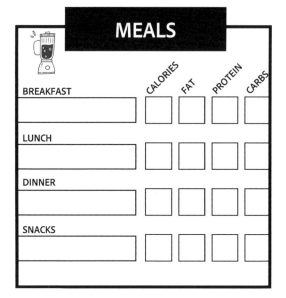

	CALORIES	FAT	PROTEIN	CARBS
BREAKFAST				
LUNCH				
DINNER				
SNACKS				

HYDRATION

🥤 🥤 🥤 🥤 🥤 🥤 🥤 🥤

SUPPLEMENTS

🙂

HOURS SLEPT LAST NIGHT

Z Z Z Z Z Z Z ✚

EXERCISE

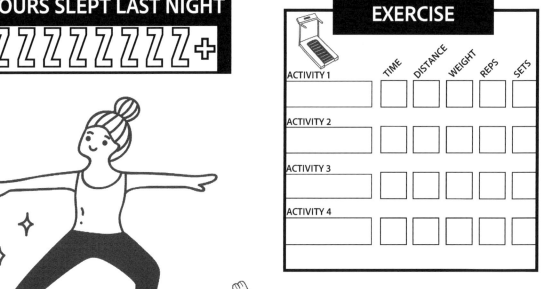

	TIME	DISTANCE	WEIGHT	REPS	SETS
ACTIVITY 1					
ACTIVITY 2					
ACTIVITY 3					
ACTIVITY 4					

Mind & Spirit

PRAYER/MEDITATION 🙏

Reflections:

_____

_____
_____
_____

SELF - CARE 🖤

I looked after me by:

_____
_____
_____
_____

GRATITUDE ⭐

I am grateful for:

_____
_____
_____
_____

TODAY I FEEL 😮 🙂 🥹 😐 😠

_____
_____

Taking Care of Body,

DATE: _____   S M T W T F S

TODAY'S GOALS

MEALS

	CALORIES	FAT	PROTEIN	CARBS
BREAKFAST				
LUNCH				
DINNER				
SNACKS				

HYDRATION

SUPPLEMENTS

:)

HOURS SLEPT LAST NIGHT

ZZZZZZZ+

EXERCISE

	TIME	DISTANCE	WEIGHT	REPS	SETS
ACTIVITY 1					
ACTIVITY 2					
ACTIVITY 3					
ACTIVITY 4					

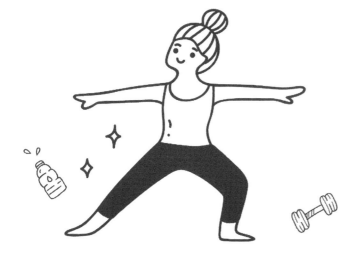

Mind & Spirit

PRAYER/MEDITATION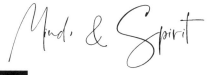

Reflections:

_____
_____
_____

SELF - CARE ♥

I looked after me by:

_____
_____
_____

GRATITUDE ✬

I am grateful for:

_____
_____
_____

TODAY I FEEL 😲 🙂 😢 😐 😠

_____
_____

Taking Care of Body,

DATE: [   ]   S M T W T F S

TODAY'S GOALS

MEALS

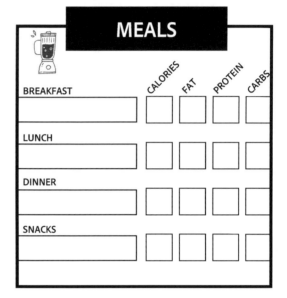

	CALORIES	FAT	PROTEIN	CARBS
BREAKFAST				
LUNCH				
DINNER				
SNACKS				

HYDRATION

SUPPLEMENTS

☺

HOURS SLEPT LAST NIGHT

Z Z Z Z Z Z Z +

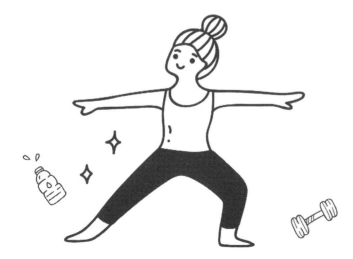

EXERCISE

	TIME	DISTANCE	WEIGHT	REPS	SETS
ACTIVITY 1					
ACTIVITY 2					
ACTIVITY 3					
ACTIVITY 4					

Mind & Spirit

PRAYER/MEDITATION 🙏

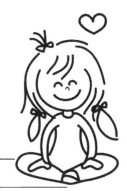

Reflections:

_____
_____
_____
_____

SELF - CARE 🖤

I looked after me by:

_____
_____
_____
_____

GRATITUDE ⭐

I am grateful for:

_____
_____
_____
_____

TODAY I FEEL 😮 🙂 😢 😐 😠

_____
_____

Taking Care of Body,

DATE: [_____]   S M T W T F S

TODAY'S GOALS

MEALS

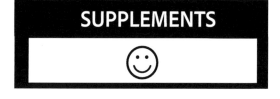

	CALORIES	FAT	PROTEIN	CARBS
BREAKFAST				
LUNCH				
DINNER				
SNACKS				

HYDRATION

SUPPLEMENTS

☺

HOURS SLEPT LAST NIGHT

ZZZZZZZ+

EXERCISE

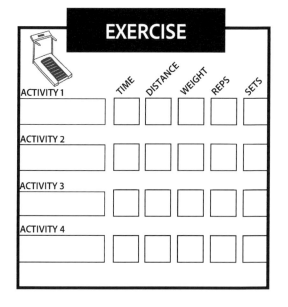

	TIME	DISTANCE	WEIGHT	REPS	SETS
ACTIVITY 1					
ACTIVITY 2					
ACTIVITY 3					
ACTIVITY 4					

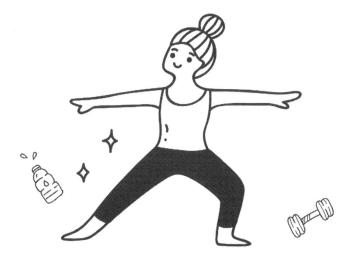

Mind & Spirit

PRAYER/MEDITATION 🙏

Reflections:

_____
_____
_____

SELF - CARE 🖤

I looked after me by:

_____
_____
_____

GRATITUDE ⭐

I am grateful for:

_____
_____
_____

TODAY I FEEL 😮 🙂 😢 😐 😠

_____
_____

Taking Care of Body.

DATE: [   ]   S M T W T F S

TODAY'S GOALS

MEALS

	CALORIES	FAT	PROTEIN	CARBS
BREAKFAST				
LUNCH				
DINNER				
SNACKS				

HYDRATION

SUPPLEMENTS

☺

HOURS SLEPT LAST NIGHT

Z Z Z Z Z Z Z +

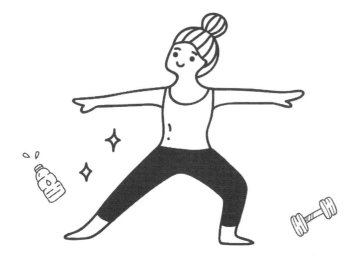

EXERCISE

	TIME	DISTANCE	WEIGHT	REPS	SETS
ACTIVITY 1					
ACTIVITY 2					
ACTIVITY 3					
ACTIVITY 4					

Mind & Spirit

PRAYER/MEDITATION 🙏

Reflections:

_____

_____

_____

_____

SELF - CARE 💙

I looked after me by:

_____

_____

_____

_____

GRATITUDE ⭐

I am grateful for:

_____

_____

_____

_____

TODAY I FEEL 😮 🙂 😢 😐 😠

_____

_____

Taking Care of Body,

DATE: _____   S M T W T F S

TODAY'S GOALS

MEALS

	CALORIES	FAT	PROTEIN	CARBS
BREAKFAST				
LUNCH				
DINNER				
SNACKS				

HYDRATION

SUPPLEMENTS

☺

HOURS SLEPT LAST NIGHT

Z Z Z Z Z Z Z +

EXERCISE

	TIME	DISTANCE	WEIGHT	REPS	SETS
ACTIVITY 1					
ACTIVITY 2					
ACTIVITY 3					
ACTIVITY 4					

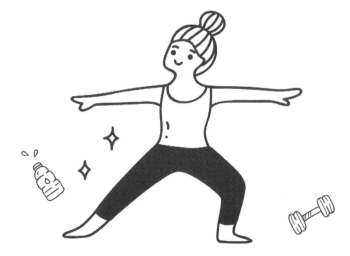

Mind & Spirit

PRAYER/MEDITATION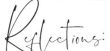

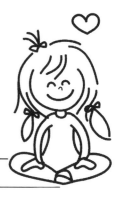

Reflections:

_____

_____

_____

SELF - CARE ♥

I looked after me by:

_____

_____

_____

GRATITUDE ✬

I am grateful for:

_____

_____

_____

TODAY I FEEL 😲 🙂 😢 😐 😠

_____

_____

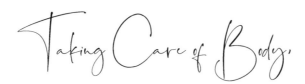

Taking Care of Body

DATE:

TODAY'S GOALS

MEALS

	CALORIES	FAT	PROTEIN	CARBS
BREAKFAST				
LUNCH				
DINNER				
SNACKS				

HYDRATION

SUPPLEMENTS

☺

HOURS SLEPT LAST NIGHT

Z Z Z Z Z Z Z +

EXERCISE

	TIME	DISTANCE	WEIGHT	REPS	SETS
ACTIVITY 1					
ACTIVITY 2					
ACTIVITY 3					
ACTIVITY 4					

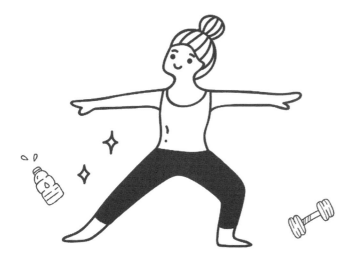

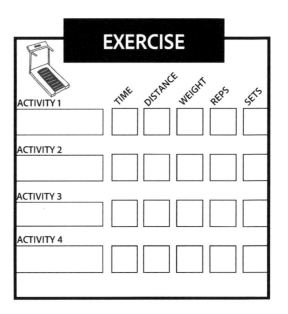

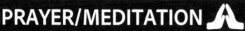 Mind & Spirit

PRAYER/MEDITATION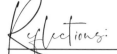

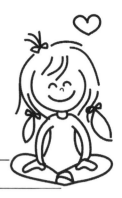

Reflections:

_____
_____
_____
_____

SELF - CARE ♥

I looked after me by:

_____
_____
_____
_____

GRATITUDE ✦

I am grateful for:

_____
_____
_____
_____

TODAY I FEEL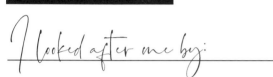

_____
_____

Taking Care of Body,

DATE: _____ S M T W T F S

TODAY'S GOALS

MEALS

	CALORIES	FAT	PROTEIN	CARBS
BREAKFAST				
LUNCH				
DINNER				
SNACKS				

HYDRATION

SUPPLEMENTS

😊

HOURS SLEPT LAST NIGHT

ZZZZZZZ+

EXERCISE

	TIME	DISTANCE	WEIGHT	REPS	SETS
ACTIVITY 1					
ACTIVITY 2					
ACTIVITY 3					
ACTIVITY 4					

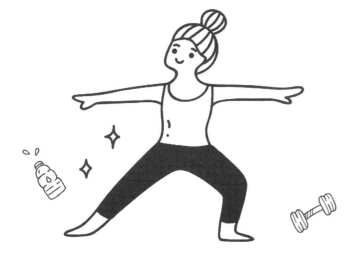

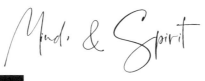

Mind & Spirit

PRAYER/MEDITATION 🙏

Reflections:

_____

_____

_____

_____

SELF - CARE 🖤

I looked after me by:

_____

_____

_____

_____

GRATITUDE ⭐

I am grateful for:

_____

_____

_____

_____

TODAY I FEEL 😮 🙂 😢 😐 😠

_____

_____

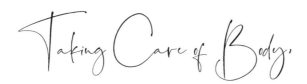

Taking Care of Body

DATE: [_____]   **S M T W T F S**

TODAY'S GOALS

MEALS

	CALORIES	FAT	PROTEIN	CARBS
BREAKFAST				
LUNCH				
DINNER				
SNACKS				

HYDRATION

SUPPLEMENTS
☺

HOURS SLEPT LAST NIGHT
Z Z Z Z Z Z Z +

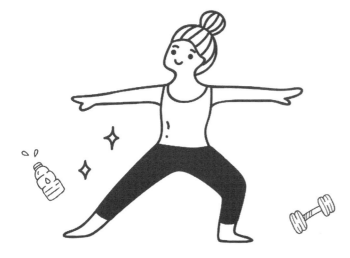

EXERCISE

	TIME	DISTANCE	WEIGHT	REPS	SETS
ACTIVITY 1					
ACTIVITY 2					
ACTIVITY 3					
ACTIVITY 4					

Mind & Spirit

PRAYER/MEDITATION 🙏

Reflections:

_____

_____

_____

SELF - CARE 🖤

I looked after me by:

_____

_____

_____

GRATITUDE ⭐

I am grateful for:

_____

_____

_____

TODAY I FEEL 😮 🙂 😢 😐 😠

_____

_____

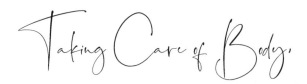

Taking Care of Body,

DATE: [_____]   S M T W T F S

TODAY'S GOALS

MEALS

	CALORIES	FAT	PROTEIN	CARBS
BREAKFAST				
LUNCH				
DINNER				
SNACKS				

HYDRATION

SUPPLEMENTS
☺

HOURS SLEPT LAST NIGHT
Z Z Z Z Z Z Z +

EXERCISE

	TIME	DISTANCE	WEIGHT	REPS	SETS
ACTIVITY 1					
ACTIVITY 2					
ACTIVITY 3					
ACTIVITY 4					

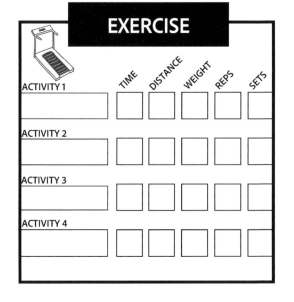

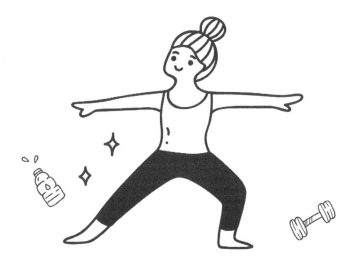

Mind & Spirit

PRAYER/MEDITATION 🙏

Reflections:

_____

_____

_____

SELF - CARE 🤍

I looked after me by:

_____

_____

_____

GRATITUDE ⭐

I am grateful for:

_____

_____

_____

TODAY I FEEL 😮 🙂 😢 😐 😠

_____

_____

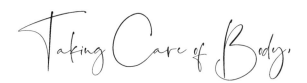

Taking Care of Body,

DATE: _____   S M T W T F S

TODAY'S GOALS

_____
_____
_____
_____
_____
_____
_____
_____

MEALS

	CALORIES	FAT	PROTEIN	CARBS
BREAKFAST				
LUNCH				
DINNER				
SNACKS				

HYDRATION

🥤 🥤 🥤 🥤 🥤 🥤 🥤 🥤

SUPPLEMENTS

☺

HOURS SLEPT LAST NIGHT

Z Z Z Z Z Z Z ✛

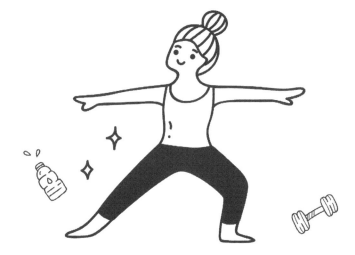

EXERCISE

	TIME	DISTANCE	WEIGHT	REPS	SETS
ACTIVITY 1					
ACTIVITY 2					
ACTIVITY 3					
ACTIVITY 4					

Mind & Spirit

PRAYER/MEDITATION

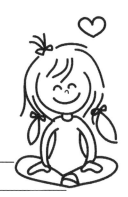

Reflections:

_____

_____

_____

SELF - CARE ♥

I looked after me by:

_____

_____

_____

GRATITUDE ✦

I am grateful for:

_____

_____

_____

TODAY I FEEL 😲 🙂 😢 😐 😠

_____

_____

Taking Care of Body.

DATE: _____ S M T W T F S

TODAY'S GOALS

MEALS

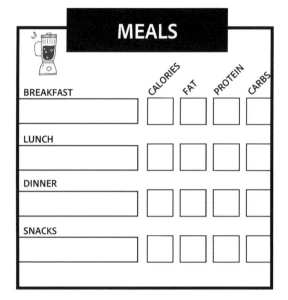

	CALORIES	FAT	PROTEIN	CARBS
BREAKFAST				
LUNCH				
DINNER				
SNACKS				

HYDRATION

SUPPLEMENTS

HOURS SLEPT LAST NIGHT

ZZZZZZZ+

EXERCISE

	TIME	DISTANCE	WEIGHT	REPS	SETS
ACTIVITY 1					
ACTIVITY 2					
ACTIVITY 3					
ACTIVITY 4					

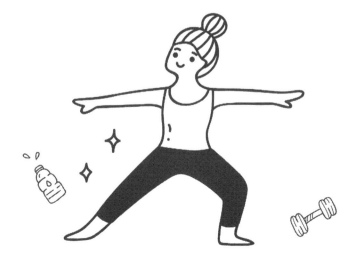

Mind & Spirit

PRAYER/MEDITATION 🙏

Reflections:

_____
_____
_____

SELF - CARE 🖤

I looked after me by:

_____
_____
_____

GRATITUDE ⭐

I am grateful for:

_____
_____
_____

TODAY I FEEL 😮 🙂 😢 😐 😠

_____
_____

Taking Care of Body,

DATE: [_____]   S M T W T F S

TODAY'S GOALS

MEALS

	CALORIES	FAT	PROTEIN	CARBS
BREAKFAST				
LUNCH				
DINNER				
SNACKS				

HYDRATION

SUPPLEMENTS

HOURS SLEPT LAST NIGHT

Z Z Z Z Z Z Z +

EXERCISE

	TIME	DISTANCE	WEIGHT	REPS	SETS
ACTIVITY 1					
ACTIVITY 2					
ACTIVITY 3					
ACTIVITY 4					

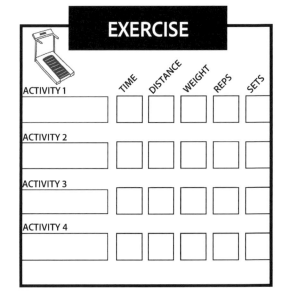

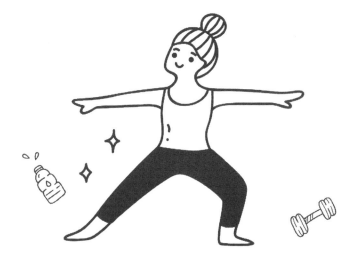

Mind & Spirit

PRAYER/MEDITATION 🙏

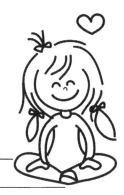

Reflections:

_____

_____

_____

_____

SELF - CARE 🖤

I looked after me by:

_____

_____

_____

_____

GRATITUDE ✫

I am grateful for:

_____

_____

_____

_____

TODAY I FEEL 😲 🙂 😢 😐 😠

_____

_____

Taking Care of Body,

DATE: _____   S M T W T F S

TODAY'S GOALS

MEALS

	CALORIES	FAT	PROTEIN	CARBS
BREAKFAST				
LUNCH				
DINNER				
SNACKS				

HYDRATION

SUPPLEMENTS

☺

HOURS SLEPT LAST NIGHT

Z Z Z Z Z Z Z +

EXERCISE

	TIME	DISTANCE	WEIGHT	REPS	SETS
ACTIVITY 1					
ACTIVITY 2					
ACTIVITY 3					
ACTIVITY 4					

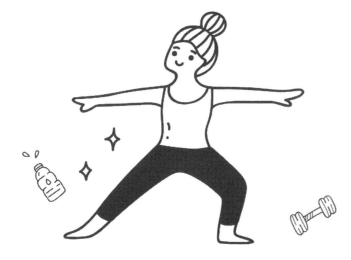

Mind & Spirit

PRAYER/MEDITATION 🙏

Reflections:

_____
_____
_____

SELF - CARE 🖤

I looked after me by:

_____
_____
_____

GRATITUDE ⭐

I am grateful for:

_____
_____
_____

TODAY I FEEL 😲 🙂 😢 😐 😠

_____
_____

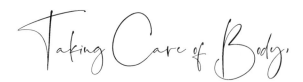

Taking Care of Body.

DATE: _____   S M T W T F S

TODAY'S GOALS

MEALS

	CALORIES	FAT	PROTEIN	CARBS
BREAKFAST				
LUNCH				
DINNER				
SNACKS				

HYDRATION

SUPPLEMENTS
☺

HOURS SLEPT LAST NIGHT
ZZZZZZZ+

EXERCISE

	TIME	DISTANCE	WEIGHT	REPS	SETS
ACTIVITY 1					
ACTIVITY 2					
ACTIVITY 3					
ACTIVITY 4					

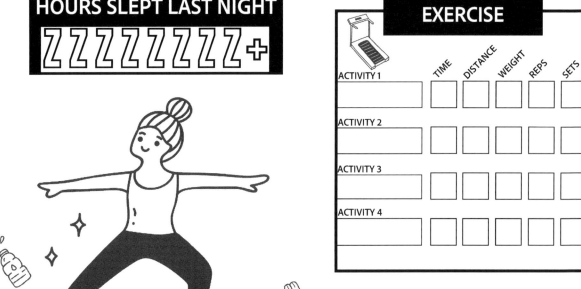

Mind & Spirit

PRAYER/MEDITATION 🙏

Reflections:

_____
_____
_____
_____

SELF - CARE 🖤

I looked after me by:

_____
_____
_____
_____

GRATITUDE ⭐

I am grateful for:

_____
_____
_____
_____

TODAY I FEEL 😲 🙂 😢 😐 😠

_____
_____

Taking Care of Body.

TODAY'S GOALS

MEALS

	CALORIES	FAT	PROTEIN	CARBS
BREAKFAST				
LUNCH				
DINNER				
SNACKS				

HYDRATION

SUPPLEMENTS

☺

HOURS SLEPT LAST NIGHT

Z Z Z Z Z Z Z +

EXERCISE

	TIME	DISTANCE	WEIGHT	REPS	SETS
ACTIVITY 1					
ACTIVITY 2					
ACTIVITY 3					
ACTIVITY 4					

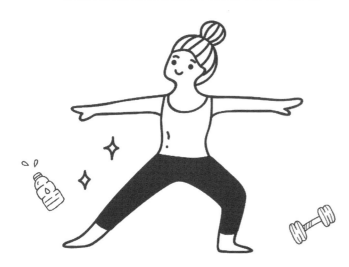

Mind & Spirit

PRAYER/MEDITATION 🙏

Reflections:

_____
_____
_____
_____

SELF - CARE 🤍

I looked after me by:

_____
_____
_____
_____

GRATITUDE ⭐

I am grateful for:

_____
_____
_____
_____

TODAY I FEEL 😮 🙂 😢 😐 😠

_____
_____

Taking Care of Body,

DATE: [_____]   S M T W T F S

TODAY'S GOALS

MEALS

	CALORIES	FAT	PROTEIN	CARBS
BREAKFAST				
LUNCH				
DINNER				
SNACKS				

HYDRATION

SUPPLEMENTS

:)

HOURS SLEPT LAST NIGHT

Z Z Z Z Z Z Z +

EXERCISE

	TIME	DISTANCE	WEIGHT	REPS	SETS
ACTIVITY 1					
ACTIVITY 2					
ACTIVITY 3					
ACTIVITY 4					

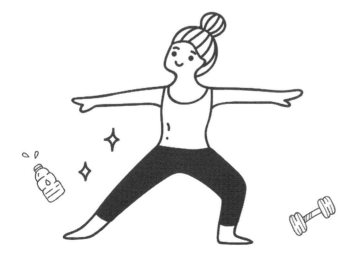

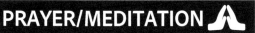

PRAYER/MEDITATION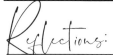

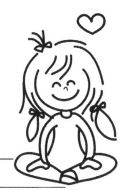

Reflections:

_____
_____
_____

SELF - CARE ♥

I looked after me by:

_____
_____
_____

GRATITUDE ⭐

I am grateful for:

_____
_____
_____

TODAY I FEEL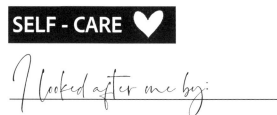

_____
_____

Taking Care of Body.

DATE: _____   S M T W T F S

TODAY'S GOALS

MEALS

	CALORIES	FAT	PROTEIN	CARBS
BREAKFAST				
LUNCH				
DINNER				
SNACKS				

HYDRATION

SUPPLEMENTS

☺

HOURS SLEPT LAST NIGHT

Z Z Z Z Z Z Z +

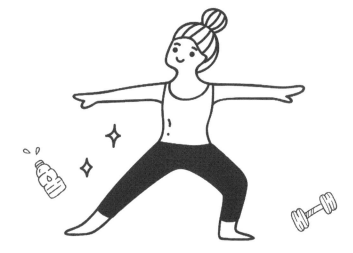

EXERCISE

	TIME	DISTANCE	WEIGHT	REPS	SETS
ACTIVITY 1					
ACTIVITY 2					
ACTIVITY 3					
ACTIVITY 4					

Mind & Spirit

PRAYER/MEDITATION 🙏

Reflections:

_____
_____
_____

SELF - CARE 🖤

I looked after me by:

_____
_____
_____

GRATITUDE ⭐

I am grateful for:

_____
_____
_____

TODAY I FEEL 😲 🙂 😢 😐 😠

_____
_____

Taking Care of Body,

DATE: _____ | S M T W T F S

TODAY'S GOALS

MEALS

	CALORIES	FAT	PROTEIN	CARBS
BREAKFAST				
LUNCH				
DINNER				
SNACKS				

HYDRATION

🥤🥤🥤🥤🥤🥤🥤🥤

SUPPLEMENTS

☺

HOURS SLEPT LAST NIGHT

Z Z Z Z Z Z Z +

EXERCISE

	TIME	DISTANCE	WEIGHT	REPS	SETS
ACTIVITY 1					
ACTIVITY 2					
ACTIVITY 3					
ACTIVITY 4					

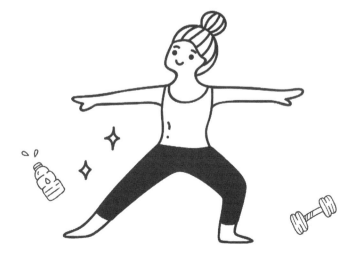

Mind & Spirit

PRAYER/MEDITATION 🙏

Reflections:

_____

_____

_____

_____

SELF - CARE 🖤

I looked after me by:

_____

_____

_____

_____

GRATITUDE ⭐

I am grateful for:

_____

_____

_____

_____

TODAY I FEEL 😮 🙂 😢 😐 😠

_____

_____

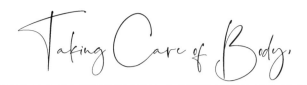

Taking Care of Body.

DATE: _____   S M T W T F S

TODAY'S GOALS

(blank lined list)

MEALS

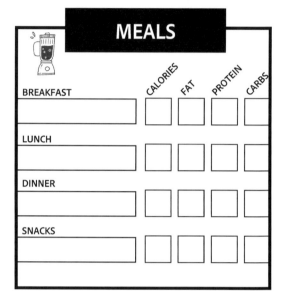

	CALORIES	FAT	PROTEIN	CARBS
BREAKFAST				
LUNCH				
DINNER				
SNACKS				

HYDRATION

(8 drink cups)

SUPPLEMENTS

☺

HOURS SLEPT LAST NIGHT

Z Z Z Z Z Z Z +

EXERCISE

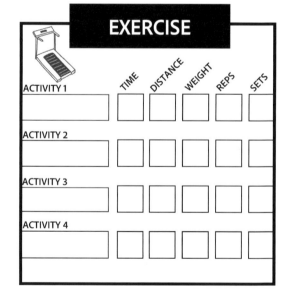

	TIME	DISTANCE	WEIGHT	REPS	SETS
ACTIVITY 1					
ACTIVITY 2					
ACTIVITY 3					
ACTIVITY 4					

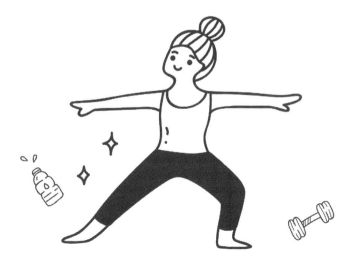

Mind & Spirit

PRAYER/MEDITATION 🙏

Reflections:

_____

_____

_____

_____

SELF - CARE ♥

I looked after me by:

_____

_____

_____

_____

GRATITUDE ⭐

I am grateful for:

_____

_____

_____

_____

TODAY I FEEL 😲 🙂 😢 😐 😠

_____

_____

Taking Care of Body.

DATE: _____   S M T W T F S

TODAY'S GOALS

MEALS

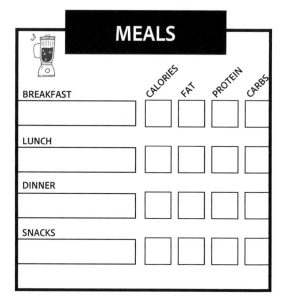

	CALORIES	FAT	PROTEIN	CARBS
BREAKFAST				
LUNCH				
DINNER				
SNACKS				

HYDRATION

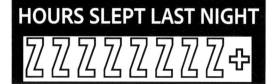

SUPPLEMENTS

☺

HOURS SLEPT LAST NIGHT

Z Z Z Z Z Z Z +

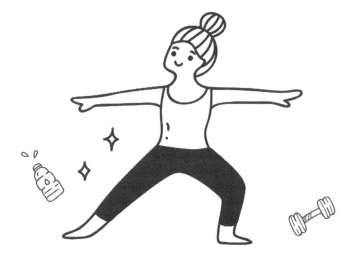

EXERCISE

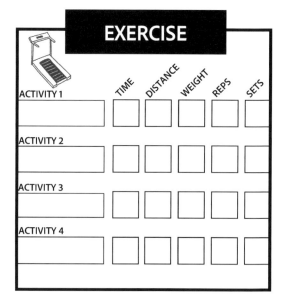

	TIME	DISTANCE	WEIGHT	REPS	SETS
ACTIVITY 1					
ACTIVITY 2					
ACTIVITY 3					
ACTIVITY 4					

Mind & Spirit

PRAYER/MEDITATION 🙏

Reflections:

_____

_____

_____

SELF - CARE 🤍

I looked after me by:

_____

_____

_____

GRATITUDE ⭐

I am grateful for:

_____

_____

_____

TODAY I FEEL 😮 🙂 😢 😐 😠

_____

_____

Taking Care of Body,

DATE: [   ]

S M T W T F S

TODAY'S GOALS

MEALS

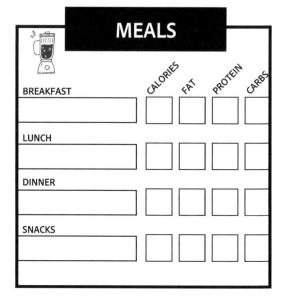

	CALORIES	FAT	PROTEIN	CARBS
BREAKFAST				
LUNCH				
DINNER				
SNACKS				

HYDRATION

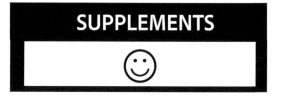

SUPPLEMENTS

☺

HOURS SLEPT LAST NIGHT

Z Z Z Z Z Z Z +

EXERCISE

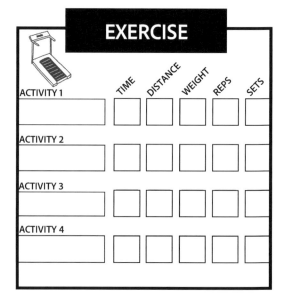

	TIME	DISTANCE	WEIGHT	REPS	SETS
ACTIVITY 1					
ACTIVITY 2					
ACTIVITY 3					
ACTIVITY 4					

Mind & Spirit

PRAYER/MEDITATION

Reflections:

_____

_____

_____

SELF - CARE

I looked after me by:

_____

_____

_____

GRATITUDE

I am grateful for:

_____

_____

_____

TODAY I FEEL

_____

_____

Taking Care of Body,

DATE: _____   S M T W T F S

TODAY'S GOALS

MEALS

	CALORIES	FAT	PROTEIN	CARBS
BREAKFAST				
LUNCH				
DINNER				
SNACKS				

HYDRATION

SUPPLEMENTS
☺

HOURS SLEPT LAST NIGHT
Z Z Z Z Z Z Z +

EXERCISE

	TIME	DISTANCE	WEIGHT	REPS	SETS
ACTIVITY 1					
ACTIVITY 2					
ACTIVITY 3					
ACTIVITY 4					

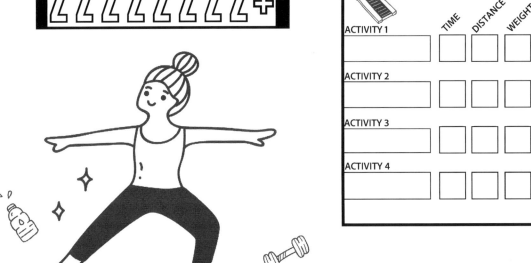

Mind & Spirit

PRAYER/MEDITATION 🙏

Reflections:

_____
_____
_____

SELF - CARE ♥

I looked after me by:

_____
_____
_____

GRATITUDE ⭐

I am grateful for:

_____
_____
_____

TODAY I FEEL 😲 🙂 😢 😐 😠

_____
_____

Taking Care of Body

DATE: _____   S M T W T F S

TODAY'S GOALS

MEALS

	CALORIES	FAT	PROTEIN	CARBS
BREAKFAST				
LUNCH				
DINNER				
SNACKS				

HYDRATION

SUPPLEMENTS

☺

HOURS SLEPT LAST NIGHT

Z Z Z Z Z Z Z +

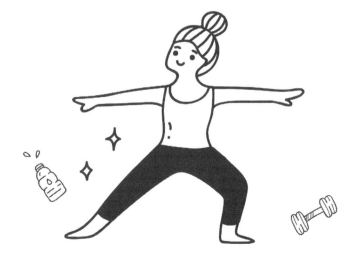

EXERCISE

	TIME	DISTANCE	WEIGHT	REPS	SETS
ACTIVITY 1					
ACTIVITY 2					
ACTIVITY 3					
ACTIVITY 4					

Mind & Spirit

PRAYER/MEDITATION 🙏

Reflections:

_____

_____

_____

SELF - CARE ♥

I looked after me by:

_____

_____

_____

GRATITUDE ⭐

I am grateful for:

_____

_____

_____

TODAY I FEEL 😮 🙂 😢 😐 😠

_____

_____

Taking Care of Body.

DATE: _____   S M T W T F S

TODAY'S GOALS

MEALS

	CALORIES	FAT	PROTEIN	CARBS
BREAKFAST				
LUNCH				
DINNER				
SNACKS				

HYDRATION

SUPPLEMENTS

☺

HOURS SLEPT LAST NIGHT

Z Z Z Z Z Z Z +

EXERCISE

	TIME	DISTANCE	WEIGHT	REPS	SETS
ACTIVITY 1					
ACTIVITY 2					
ACTIVITY 3					
ACTIVITY 4					

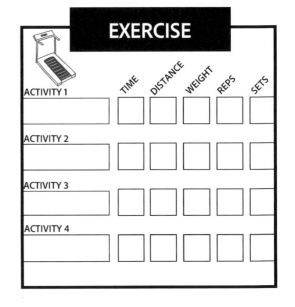

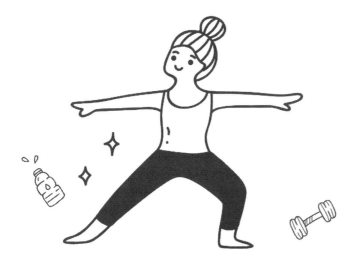

Mind & Spirit

PRAYER/MEDITATION 🙏

Reflections:

_____
_____
_____
_____

SELF - CARE 🖤

I looked after me by:

_____
_____
_____
_____

GRATITUDE ⭐

I am grateful for:

_____
_____
_____
_____

TODAY I FEEL 😮 🙂 😢 😐 😠

_____
_____

Taking Care of Body.

TODAY'S GOALS

MEALS

	CALORIES	FAT	PROTEIN	CARBS
BREAKFAST				
LUNCH				
DINNER				
SNACKS				

HYDRATION

SUPPLEMENTS

☺

HOURS SLEPT LAST NIGHT

ZZZZZZZ+

EXERCISE

	TIME	DISTANCE	WEIGHT	REPS	SETS
ACTIVITY 1					
ACTIVITY 2					
ACTIVITY 3					
ACTIVITY 4					

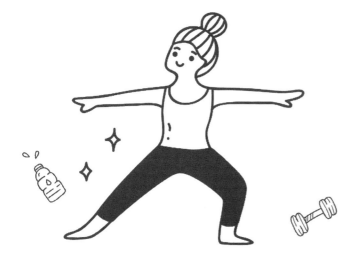

Mind, & Spirit

PRAYER/MEDITATION 🙏

Reflections:

_____

_____

_____

SELF - CARE 🖤

I looked after me by:

_____

_____

_____

GRATITUDE ⭐

I am grateful for:

_____

_____

_____

TODAY I FEEL 😮 🙂 😢 😐 😠

_____

_____

Taking Care of Body,

DATE: _____   S M T W T F S

TODAY'S GOALS

MEALS

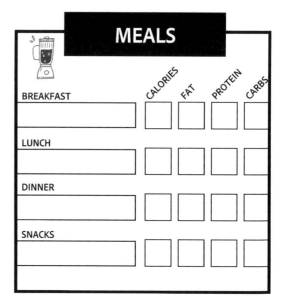

	CALORIES	FAT	PROTEIN	CARBS
BREAKFAST				
LUNCH				
DINNER				
SNACKS				

HYDRATION

SUPPLEMENTS

☺

HOURS SLEPT LAST NIGHT

Z Z Z Z Z Z Z +

EXERCISE

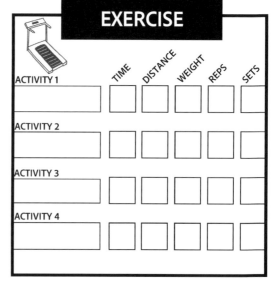

	TIME	DISTANCE	WEIGHT	REPS	SETS
ACTIVITY 1					
ACTIVITY 2					
ACTIVITY 3					
ACTIVITY 4					

Mind & Spirit

PRAYER/MEDITATION 🙏

Reflections:

_____

_____

_____

SELF - CARE 💙

I looked after me by:

_____

_____

_____

GRATITUDE ⭐

I am grateful for:

_____

_____

_____

TODAY I FEEL 😮 🙂 😢 😐 😠

_____

_____

Taking Care of Body,

DATE: [   ]   S M T W T F S

TODAY'S GOALS

MEALS

	CALORIES	FAT	PROTEIN	CARBS
BREAKFAST				
LUNCH				
DINNER				
SNACKS				

HYDRATION

SUPPLEMENTS

☺

HOURS SLEPT LAST NIGHT

ZZZZZZZ+

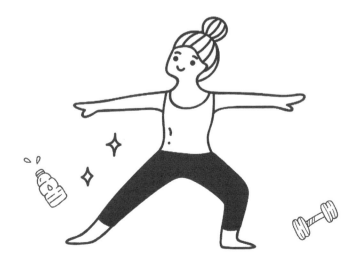

EXERCISE

	TIME	DISTANCE	WEIGHT	REPS	SETS
ACTIVITY 1					
ACTIVITY 2					
ACTIVITY 3					
ACTIVITY 4					

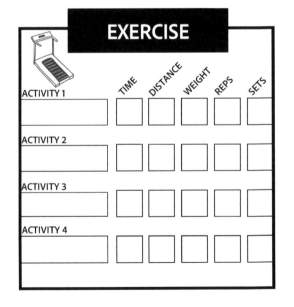

Mind & Spirit

PRAYER/MEDITATION 🙏

Reflections:

_____
_____
_____
_____

SELF - CARE 🖤

I looked after me by:

_____
_____
_____
_____

GRATITUDE ⭐

I am grateful for:

_____
_____
_____
_____

TODAY I FEEL 😲 🙂 😢 😐 😠

_____
_____

Taking Care of Body,

DATE: _____   S M T W T F S

TODAY'S GOALS

MEALS

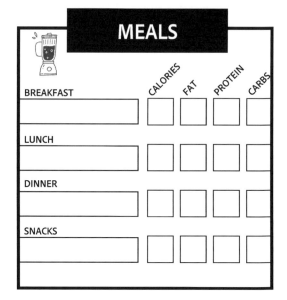

BREAKFAST	CALORIES	FAT	PROTEIN	CARBS
LUNCH				
DINNER				
SNACKS				

HYDRATION

SUPPLEMENTS

☺

HOURS SLEPT LAST NIGHT

Z Z Z Z Z Z Z +

EXERCISE

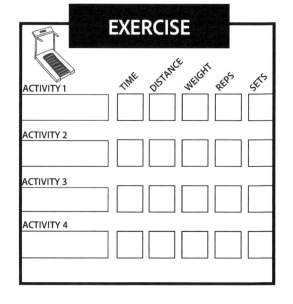

	TIME	DISTANCE	WEIGHT	REPS	SETS
ACTIVITY 1					
ACTIVITY 2					
ACTIVITY 3					
ACTIVITY 4					

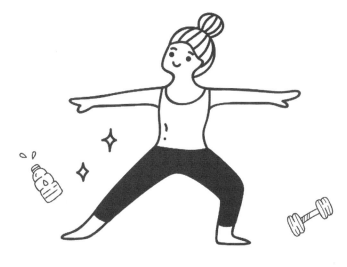

Mind & Spirit

PRAYER/MEDITATION 🙏

Reflections:

_____
_____
_____
_____

SELF - CARE ♥

I looked after me by:

_____
_____
_____
_____

GRATITUDE ⭐

I am grateful for:

_____
_____
_____
_____

TODAY I FEEL 😮 🙂 🥲 😐 😠

_____
_____

Taking Care of Body.

DATE: [   ]   S M T W T F S

TODAY'S GOALS

MEALS

	CALORIES	FAT	PROTEIN	CARBS
BREAKFAST				
LUNCH				
DINNER				
SNACKS				

HYDRATION

SUPPLEMENTS
☺

HOURS SLEPT LAST NIGHT
ZZZZZZZ+

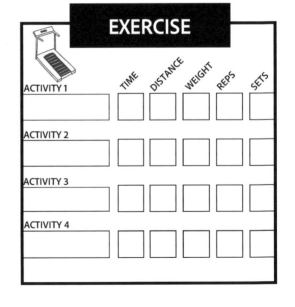

EXERCISE

	TIME	DISTANCE	WEIGHT	REPS	SETS
ACTIVITY 1					
ACTIVITY 2					
ACTIVITY 3					
ACTIVITY 4					

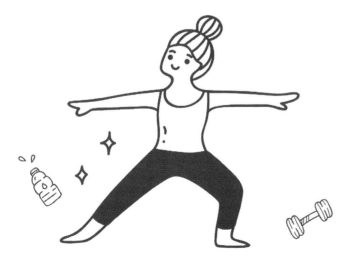

Mind & Spirit

PRAYER/MEDITATION 🙏

Reflections:

_____

_____

_____

SELF - CARE 🤍

I looked after me by:

_____

_____

_____

GRATITUDE ⭐

I am grateful for:

_____

_____

_____

TODAY I FEEL 😮 🙂 😢 😐 😠

_____

_____

Taking Care of Body,

DATE: _____   S M T W T F S

TODAY'S GOALS

MEALS

	CALORIES	FAT	PROTEIN	CARBS
BREAKFAST				
LUNCH				
DINNER				
SNACKS				

HYDRATION

SUPPLEMENTS

☺

HOURS SLEPT LAST NIGHT

Z Z Z Z Z Z Z +

EXERCISE

	TIME	DISTANCE	WEIGHT	REPS	SETS
ACTIVITY 1					
ACTIVITY 2					
ACTIVITY 3					
ACTIVITY 4					

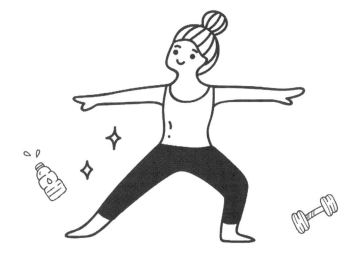

Mind & Spirit

PRAYER/MEDITATION 🙏

Reflections:

_____

_____

_____

SELF - CARE 🖤

I looked after me by:

_____

_____

_____

GRATITUDE ⭐

I am grateful for:

_____

_____

_____

TODAY I FEEL 😲 🙂 😢 😐 😠

_____

_____

Taking Care of Body.

DATE: _____   S M T W T F S

TODAY'S GOALS

MEALS

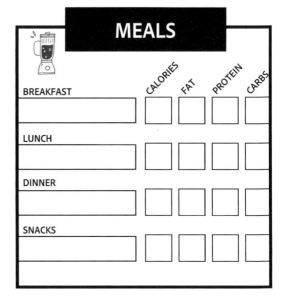

	CALORIES	FAT	PROTEIN	CARBS
BREAKFAST				
LUNCH				
DINNER				
SNACKS				

HYDRATION

SUPPLEMENTS

☺

HOURS SLEPT LAST NIGHT

ZZZZZZZ+

EXERCISE

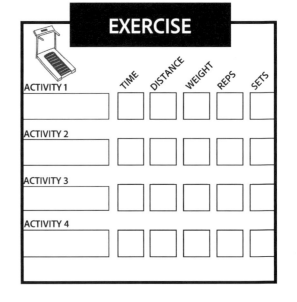

	TIME	DISTANCE	WEIGHT	REPS	SETS
ACTIVITY 1					
ACTIVITY 2					
ACTIVITY 3					
ACTIVITY 4					

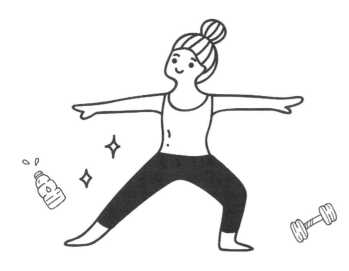

Mind & Spirit

PRAYER/MEDITATION 🙏

Reflections:

_____

_____

_____

SELF - CARE 🖤

I looked after me by:

_____

_____

_____

GRATITUDE ⭐

I am grateful for:

_____

_____

_____

TODAY I FEEL 😮 🙂 😢 😐 😠

_____

_____

Taking Care of Body,

DATE: _____   S M T W T F S

TODAY'S GOALS

MEALS

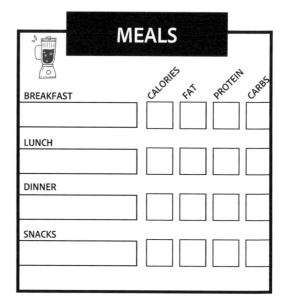

	CALORIES	FAT	PROTEIN	CARBS
BREAKFAST				
LUNCH				
DINNER				
SNACKS				

HYDRATION

SUPPLEMENTS

☺

HOURS SLEPT LAST NIGHT

ZZZZZZZ+

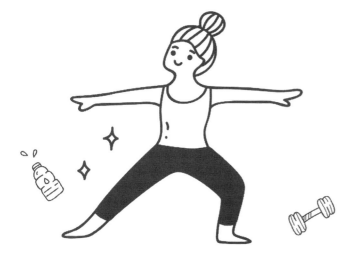

EXERCISE

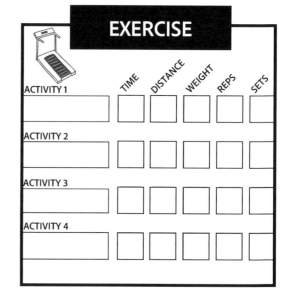

	TIME	DISTANCE	WEIGHT	REPS	SETS
ACTIVITY 1					
ACTIVITY 2					
ACTIVITY 3					
ACTIVITY 4					

Mind & Spirit

PRAYER/MEDITATION 🙏

Reflections:

_____
_____
_____
_____

SELF - CARE 🖤

I looked after me by:

_____
_____
_____

GRATITUDE ⭐

I am grateful for:

_____
_____
_____

TODAY I FEEL 😲 🙂 😢 😐 😠

_____
_____

Taking Care of Body,

DATE: _____   S M T W T F S

TODAY'S GOALS

MEALS

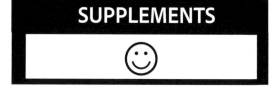

	CALORIES	FAT	PROTEIN	CARBS
BREAKFAST				
LUNCH				
DINNER				
SNACKS				

HYDRATION

SUPPLEMENTS

☺

HOURS SLEPT LAST NIGHT

Z Z Z Z Z Z Z +

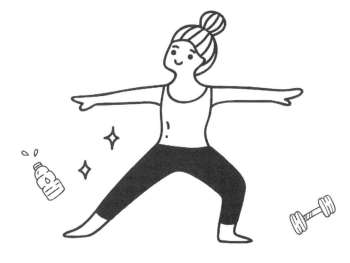

EXERCISE

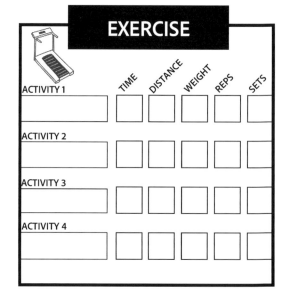

	TIME	DISTANCE	WEIGHT	REPS	SETS
ACTIVITY 1					
ACTIVITY 2					
ACTIVITY 3					
ACTIVITY 4					

Mind & Spirit

PRAYER/MEDITATION 🙏

Reflections:

_____

_____

_____

SELF - CARE 🖤

I looked after me by:

_____

_____

_____

GRATITUDE ⭐

I am grateful for:

_____

_____

_____

TODAY I FEEL 😲 🙂 😢 😐 😠

_____

_____

Taking Care of Body,

DATE: _____   S M T W T F S

TODAY'S GOALS

MEALS

	CALORIES	FAT	PROTEIN	CARBS
BREAKFAST				
LUNCH				
DINNER				
SNACKS				

HYDRATION

SUPPLEMENTS

☺

HOURS SLEPT LAST NIGHT

Z Z Z Z Z Z Z +

EXERCISE

	TIME	DISTANCE	WEIGHT	REPS	SETS
ACTIVITY 1					
ACTIVITY 2					
ACTIVITY 3					
ACTIVITY 4					

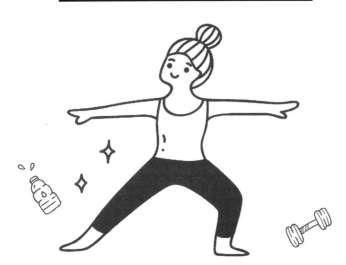

Mind & Spirit

PRAYER/MEDITATION 🙏

Reflections:

_____

_____

_____

SELF - CARE ♥

I looked after me by:

_____

_____

_____

GRATITUDE ⭐

I am grateful for:

_____

_____

_____

TODAY I FEEL 😮 🙂 😢 😐 😠

_____

_____

Taking Care of Body,

DATE: _____   **S M T W T F S**

TODAY'S GOALS

MEALS

	CALORIES	FAT	PROTEIN	CARBS
BREAKFAST				
LUNCH				
DINNER				
SNACKS				

HYDRATION

SUPPLEMENTS

☺

HOURS SLEPT LAST NIGHT

Z Z Z Z Z Z Z +

EXERCISE

	TIME	DISTANCE	WEIGHT	REPS	SETS
ACTIVITY 1					
ACTIVITY 2					
ACTIVITY 3					
ACTIVITY 4					

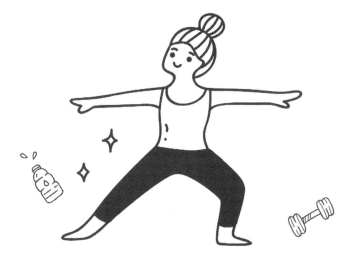

Mind & Spirit

PRAYER/MEDITATION 🙏

Reflections:

_____

_____

_____

SELF - CARE 🖤

I looked after me by:

_____

_____

_____

GRATITUDE ⭐

I am grateful for:

_____

_____

_____

TODAY I FEEL 😲 🙂 😢 😐 😠

_____

_____

Taking Care of Body.

DATE: _____   S M T W T F S

TODAY'S GOALS

MEALS

	CALORIES	FAT	PROTEIN	CARBS
BREAKFAST				
LUNCH				
DINNER				
SNACKS				

HYDRATION

SUPPLEMENTS

☺

HOURS SLEPT LAST NIGHT

Z Z Z Z Z Z Z +

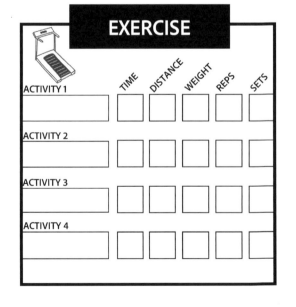

EXERCISE

	TIME	DISTANCE	WEIGHT	REPS	SETS
ACTIVITY 1					
ACTIVITY 2					
ACTIVITY 3					
ACTIVITY 4					

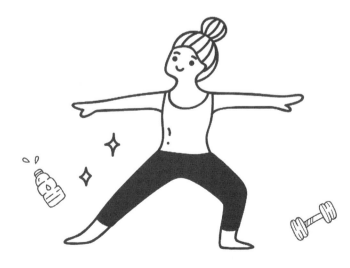

Mind & Spirit

PRAYER/MEDITATION 🙏

Reflections:

_____

_____

_____

SELF - CARE 🖤

I looked after me by:

_____

_____

_____

GRATITUDE ⭐

I am grateful for:

_____

_____

_____

TODAY I FEEL 😲 🙂 😢 😐 😠

_____

_____

Taking Care of Body,

DATE: [_____]   S M T W T F S

TODAY'S GOALS

MEALS

	CALORIES	FAT	PROTEIN	CARBS
BREAKFAST				
LUNCH				
DINNER				
SNACKS				

HYDRATION

🥤 🥤 🥤 🥤 🥤 🥤 🥤 🥤

SUPPLEMENTS

☺

HOURS SLEPT LAST NIGHT

Z Z Z Z Z Z Z +

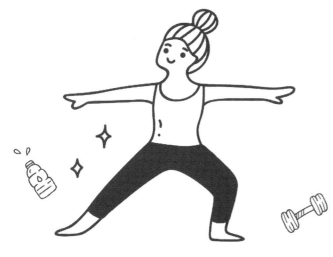

EXERCISE

	TIME	DISTANCE	WEIGHT	REPS	SETS
ACTIVITY 1					
ACTIVITY 2					
ACTIVITY 3					
ACTIVITY 4					

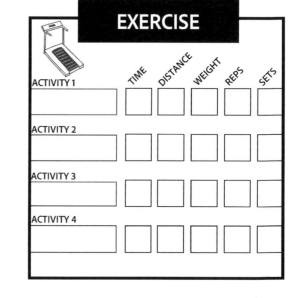

Mind & Spirit

PRAYER/MEDITATION 🙏

Reflections:

_____

_____

_____

SELF - CARE 🖤

I looked after me by:

_____

_____

_____

GRATITUDE ⭐

I am grateful for:

_____

_____

_____

TODAY I FEEL 😲 🙂 😢 😐 😠

_____

_____

Taking Care of Body,

DATE: _____   S M T W T F S

TODAY'S GOALS

MEALS

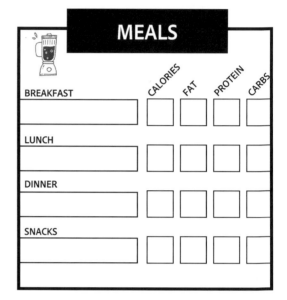

	CALORIES	FAT	PROTEIN	CARBS
BREAKFAST				
LUNCH				
DINNER				
SNACKS				

HYDRATION

SUPPLEMENTS

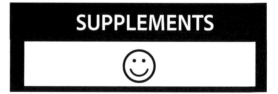

HOURS SLEPT LAST NIGHT

ZZZZZZZ+

EXERCISE

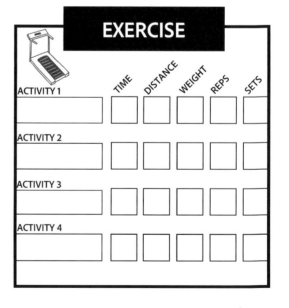

	TIME	DISTANCE	WEIGHT	REPS	SETS
ACTIVITY 1					
ACTIVITY 2					
ACTIVITY 3					
ACTIVITY 4					

Mind & Spirit

PRAYER/MEDITATION 🙏

Reflections:

_____

_____

_____

_____

SELF - CARE 💙

I looked after me by:

_____

_____

_____

_____

GRATITUDE ⭐

I am grateful for:

_____

_____

_____

_____

TODAY I FEEL 😲 🙂 😢 😐 😠

_____

_____

Taking Care of Body,

DATE: [　　　　　　　]   S M T W T F S

TODAY'S GOALS

MEALS

	CALORIES	FAT	PROTEIN	CARBS
BREAKFAST				
LUNCH				
DINNER				
SNACKS				

HYDRATION

SUPPLEMENTS

:)

HOURS SLEPT LAST NIGHT

ZZZZZZZ+

EXERCISE

	TIME	DISTANCE	WEIGHT	REPS	SETS
ACTIVITY 1					
ACTIVITY 2					
ACTIVITY 3					
ACTIVITY 4					

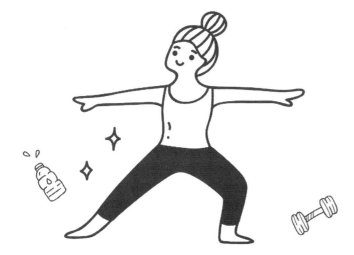

Mind & Spirit

PRAYER/MEDITATION 🙏

Reflections:

_____

_____

_____

SELF - CARE 🖤

I looked after me by:

_____

_____

_____

GRATITUDE ⭐

I am grateful for:

_____

_____

_____

TODAY I FEEL 😮 🙂 😢 😐 😠

_____

_____

Taking Care of Body

DATE: [   ]   S M T W T F S

TODAY'S GOALS

MEALS

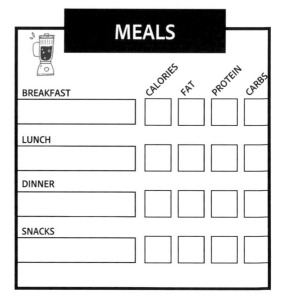

	CALORIES	FAT	PROTEIN	CARBS
BREAKFAST				
LUNCH				
DINNER				
SNACKS				

HYDRATION

🥤 🥤 🥤 🥤 🥤 🥤 🥤 🥤

SUPPLEMENTS

☺

HOURS SLEPT LAST NIGHT

Z Z Z Z Z Z Z +

EXERCISE

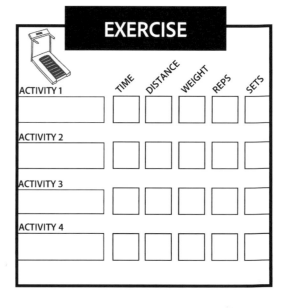

	TIME	DISTANCE	WEIGHT	REPS	SETS
ACTIVITY 1					
ACTIVITY 2					
ACTIVITY 3					
ACTIVITY 4					

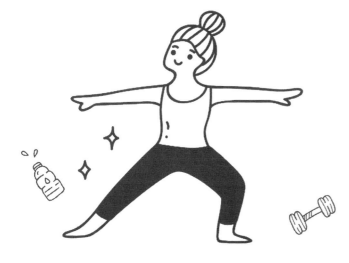

Mind & Spirit

PRAYER/MEDITATION

Reflections:

_____
_____
_____

SELF - CARE ♥

I looked after me by:

_____
_____
_____

GRATITUDE ✮

I am grateful for:

_____
_____
_____

TODAY I FEEL 😲 🙂 😢 😐 😠

_____
_____

Taking Care of Body

DATE: _____   S M T W T F S

TODAY'S GOALS

MEALS

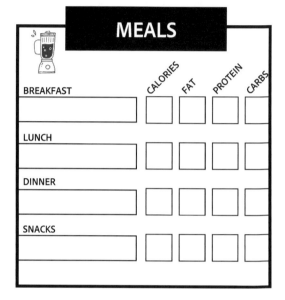

	CALORIES	FAT	PROTEIN	CARBS
BREAKFAST				
LUNCH				
DINNER				
SNACKS				

HYDRATION

SUPPLEMENTS

☺

HOURS SLEPT LAST NIGHT

ZZZZZZZ+

EXERCISE

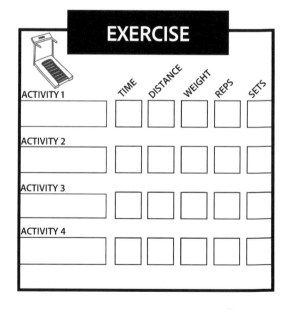

	TIME	DISTANCE	WEIGHT	REPS	SETS
ACTIVITY 1					
ACTIVITY 2					
ACTIVITY 3					
ACTIVITY 4					

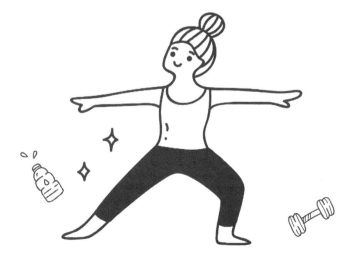

Mind & Spirit

PRAYER/MEDITATION 🙏

Reflections:

_____
_____
_____
_____

SELF - CARE 🖤

I looked after me by:

_____
_____
_____
_____

GRATITUDE ⭐

I am grateful for:

_____
_____
_____
_____

TODAY I FEEL 😮 🙂 😢 😐 😠

_____
_____

Taking Care of Body

DATE: _____   **S M T W T F S**

TODAY'S GOALS

MEALS

	CALORIES	FAT	PROTEIN	CARBS
BREAKFAST				
LUNCH				
DINNER				
SNACKS				

HYDRATION

SUPPLEMENTS

☺

HOURS SLEPT LAST NIGHT

Z Z Z Z Z Z Z +

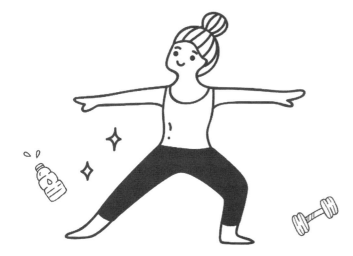

EXERCISE

	TIME	DISTANCE	WEIGHT	REPS	SETS
ACTIVITY 1					
ACTIVITY 2					
ACTIVITY 3					
ACTIVITY 4					

Mind & Spirit

PRAYER/MEDITATION 🙏

Reflections:

_____

_____

_____

SELF - CARE 🖤

I looked after me by:

_____

_____

_____

GRATITUDE ⭐

I am grateful for:

_____

_____

_____

TODAY I FEEL 😲 🙂 😢 😐 😠

_____

_____

Taking Care of Body,

DATE: _____   S M T W T F S

TODAY'S GOALS

MEALS

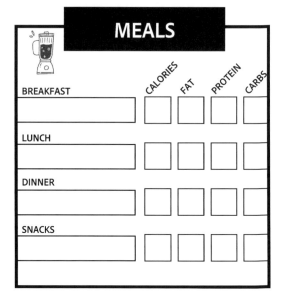

	CALORIES	FAT	PROTEIN	CARBS
BREAKFAST				
LUNCH				
DINNER				
SNACKS				

HYDRATION

SUPPLEMENTS

HOURS SLEPT LAST NIGHT

Z Z Z Z Z Z Z +

EXERCISE

	TIME	DISTANCE	WEIGHT	REPS	SETS
ACTIVITY 1					
ACTIVITY 2					
ACTIVITY 3					
ACTIVITY 4					

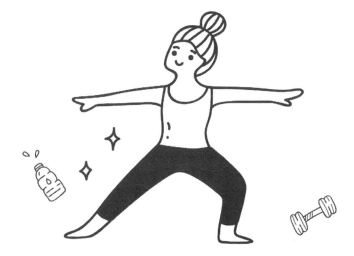

Mind & Spirit

PRAYER/MEDITATION 🙏

Reflections:

_____
_____
_____

SELF - CARE 💜

I looked after me by:

_____
_____
_____

GRATITUDE ⭐

I am grateful for:

_____
_____
_____

TODAY I FEEL 😮 🙂 😢 😐 😠

_____
_____

Taking Care of Body

DATE: _____   S M T W T F S

TODAY'S GOALS

MEALS

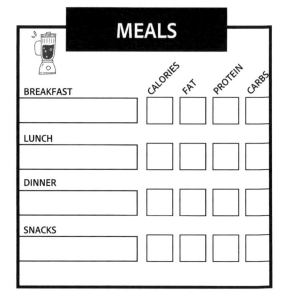

	CALORIES	FAT	PROTEIN	CARBS
BREAKFAST				
LUNCH				
DINNER				
SNACKS				

HYDRATION

🥤 🥤 🥤 🥤 🥤 🥤 🥤 🥤

SUPPLEMENTS

🙂

HOURS SLEPT LAST NIGHT

Z Z Z Z Z Z Z +

EXERCISE

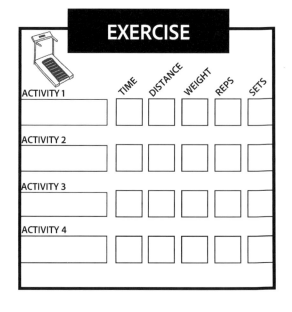

	TIME	DISTANCE	WEIGHT	REPS	SETS
ACTIVITY 1					
ACTIVITY 2					
ACTIVITY 3					
ACTIVITY 4					

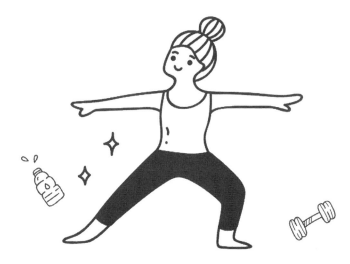

Mind & Spirit

PRAYER/MEDITATION 🙏

Reflections:

_____

_____

_____

SELF - CARE 🖤

I looked after me by:

_____

_____

_____

GRATITUDE ⭐

I am grateful for:

_____

_____

_____

TODAY I FEEL 😮 🙂 😢 😐 😠

_____

_____

Taking Care of Body

DATE: _____   S M T W T F S

TODAY'S GOALS

MEALS

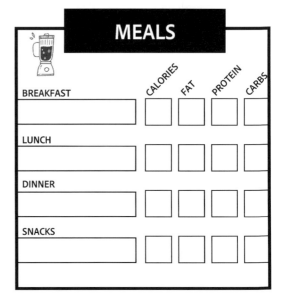

	CALORIES	FAT	PROTEIN	CARBS
BREAKFAST				
LUNCH				
DINNER				
SNACKS				

HYDRATION

SUPPLEMENTS

HOURS SLEPT LAST NIGHT

ZZZZZZZ+

EXERCISE

	TIME	DISTANCE	WEIGHT	REPS	SETS
ACTIVITY 1					
ACTIVITY 2					
ACTIVITY 3					
ACTIVITY 4					

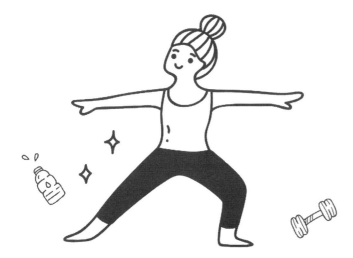

Mind & Spirit

PRAYER/MEDITATION 🙏

Reflections:

_____
_____
_____

SELF - CARE 🖤

I looked after me by:

_____
_____
_____

GRATITUDE ⭐

I am grateful for:

_____
_____
_____

TODAY I FEEL 😲 🙂 😢 😐 😠

_____
_____

Taking Care of Body

DATE: [   ]   S M T W T F S

TODAY'S GOALS

MEALS

	CALORIES	FAT	PROTEIN	CARBS
BREAKFAST				
LUNCH				
DINNER				
SNACKS				

HYDRATION

SUPPLEMENTS
☺

HOURS SLEPT LAST NIGHT
Z Z Z Z Z Z Z +

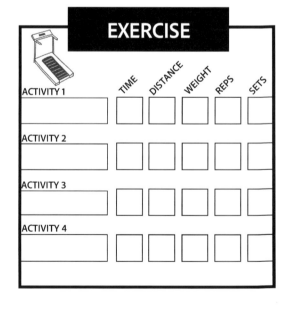

EXERCISE

	TIME	DISTANCE	WEIGHT	REPS	SETS
ACTIVITY 1					
ACTIVITY 2					
ACTIVITY 3					
ACTIVITY 4					

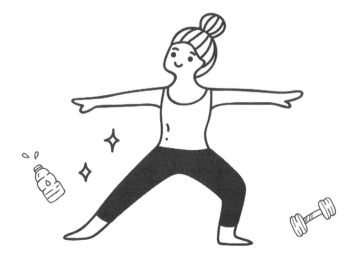

Mind, & Spirit

PRAYER/MEDITATION 🙏

Reflections:

_____

_____

_____

SELF - CARE 🖤

I looked after me by:

_____

_____

_____

GRATITUDE ⭐

I am grateful for:

_____

_____

_____

TODAY I FEEL 😮 🙂 😢 😐 😠

_____

_____

Taking Care of Body,

DATE: [_____]   **S M T W T F S**

TODAY'S GOALS

MEALS

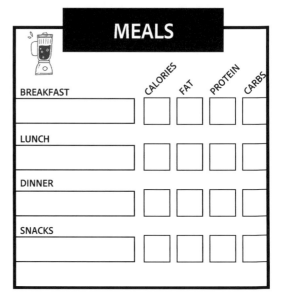

	CALORIES	FAT	PROTEIN	CARBS
BREAKFAST				
LUNCH				
DINNER				
SNACKS				

HYDRATION

🥤 🥤 🥤 🥤 🥤 🥤 🥤 🥤

SUPPLEMENTS

☺

HOURS SLEPT LAST NIGHT

Z Z Z Z Z Z Z +

EXERCISE

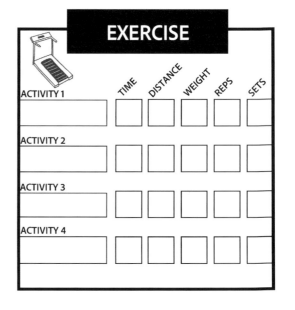

	TIME	DISTANCE	WEIGHT	REPS	SETS
ACTIVITY 1					
ACTIVITY 2					
ACTIVITY 3					
ACTIVITY 4					

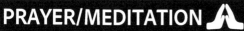

PRAYER/MEDITATION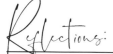

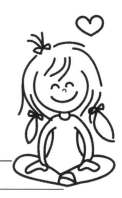

Reflections:

_____

_____

_____

SELF - CARE ♥

I looked after me by:

_____

_____

_____

GRATITUDE ⭐

I am grateful for:

_____

_____

_____

TODAY I FEEL 😮 🙂 😢 😐 😠

_____

_____

Taking Care of Body

DATE: [   ]   S M T W T F S

TODAY'S GOALS

MEALS

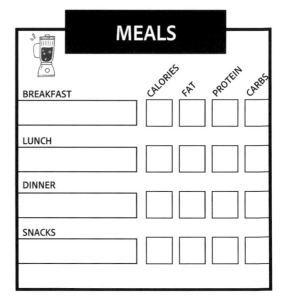

	CALORIES	FAT	PROTEIN	CARBS
BREAKFAST				
LUNCH				
DINNER				
SNACKS				

HYDRATION

SUPPLEMENTS

HOURS SLEPT LAST NIGHT

ZZZZZZZ+

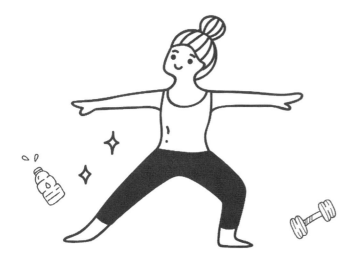

EXERCISE

	TIME	DISTANCE	WEIGHT	REPS	SETS
ACTIVITY 1					
ACTIVITY 2					
ACTIVITY 3					
ACTIVITY 4					

Made in United States
Orlando, FL
13 March 2022

15750123R10204